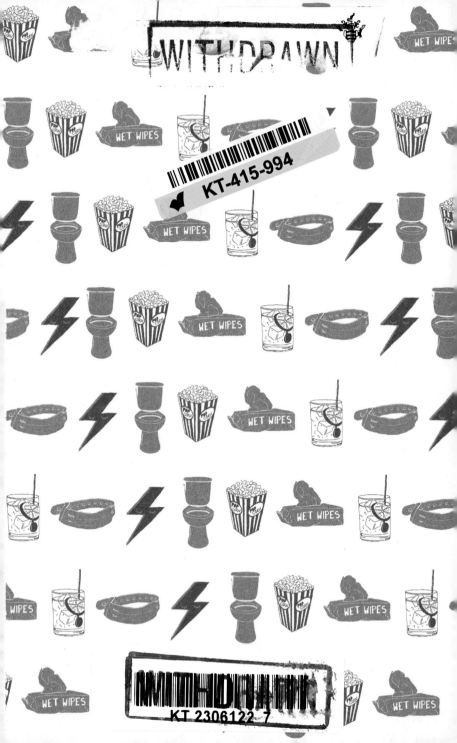

'What a refreshingly honest account of life with Crohn's disease. As a Crohn's sufferer you will find yourself nodding as you turn the pages through many experiences that we have all gone through. [Kathleen's] wit and sense of humour shines through to make it an enjoyable read, and it is no small achievement to make such a tough topic light-hearted. I think this book could be enjoyed by those newly diagnosed, or who have suffered for many years.'

— Sally Cooney, Patient Ambassador, forCrohns

'Kathleen works wonders as a funny, strong, and honest guide to living with Crohn's disease. *Go Your Crohn Way* is undeniably humane and handy.'

— Ken Baumann, Author and Publisher

'Crystal-clear, dead-solid accurate and witty explanations typify this book. Whether you are a new Crohn's patient, a friend or relative of a patient, or even a 30-year old Crohn's Disease patient like me, you will enjoy the compressive wisdom gained by reading *Go Your Crohn Way*.'

— Michael A. Weiss, Esq., MBA,
Founder of Crohn's Disease Warrior Patrol
and Professional Patient Perspective

GO YOUR CROHN WAY

of related interest

The Mystery of Pain
Douglas Nelson
ISBN 978 1 84819 152 5
eISBN 978 0 85701 116 9

Pain is Really Strange
Steve Haines
Art by Sophie Standing
ISBN 978 1 84819 264 5
eISBN 978 0 85701 212 8
Part of the …is Really Strange *Series*

GO YOUR CROHN WAY

A GUTSY GUIDE TO LIVING WITH CROHN'S DISEASE

KATHLEEN NICHOLLS

SINGING
DRAGON
LONDON AND PHILADELPHIA

www.singingdragon.com

Library of Congress Cataloging in Publication Data
Names: Nicholls, Kathleen D., author.
Title: Go your Crohn way : a gutsy guide to living with Crohn's disease /
Kathleen Nicholls ; illustrated by Kara McHale.
Description: London ; Philadelphia : Singing Dragon, 2016.
Identifiers: LCCN 2015047588 | ISBN 9781848193161 (alk. paper)
Subjects: LCSH: Crohn's disease--Popular works. | Health--Popular works. |
Wit and humor--Psychological aspects.
Classification: LCC RC862.E52 N53 2016 | DDC 616.3/44--
dc23 LC record available at http://lccn.loc.gov/2015047588

British Library Cataloguing in Publication Data
A CIP catalogue record for this book is available from the British Library

ISBN 978 1 84819 316 1
eISBN 978 0 85701 268 5

Printed and bound in Great Britain

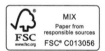

FOR JAMES,
FOR KATHLEEN AND RICHARD,
FOR WET WIPES.

CONTENTS

FOUR WORD(S)

I HAVE CROHN'S DISEASE

Before I begin, let me make one thing crystal clear. This is NOT a self-help book.

'Self-help' is a redundant phrase to me in itself, as by definition you aren't 'helping' yourself, you are picking up a book and hoping it will tell you what to do next. I can't, and won't, offer you that luxury.

I wouldn't be so confident as to even know where to start.

Crohn's as an illness is so unusual, yet so oddly unique, that everyone who experiences it suffers differently. That's why I just can't accept the idea that there is one solution for all. One coping mechanism does not fit everyone.

I am just a woman. A diseased woman, standing in front of you, asking you to love her. No, of course not, you're already there, right?

I cannot tell you what to eat or drink to make you feel a little better. I can't wave a magic wand made of the written word to ease your weary mind and I certainly can't *cure* your disease. I'd absolutely *love* to have the power to do all of the above, but like I said, I'm just a woman.

I can, however, promise to give you a few solid pages of ups and downs, insight and hints and tips in living with a chronic illness. Doesn't sound like much I suppose, but hey, I'm no miracle worker.

I simply aim to show you, through sharing my own experiences, that there is life beyond an incurable illness. That life can be as full to the brim of fun and happiness as you want it to be.

I'm not deluded; there is no great glory and certainly no pleasure in having Crohn's Disease. It's HARD and unfair and really disheartening at times. I only intend to share with you my story in the hope that you can begin to see past the negative aspects and look to your future without bitterness and anger. That may take days, months or even years in living with the condition, but I hope we'll get a little closer to the edge of that particular map by the end of this volume.

I've been a Crohn's patient for several years. I've endured more treatments and sampled more medication than I can reasonably count and had (so far) only one major operation. That operation, thankfully, saved my life and allowed *you* the privilege of reading this humble tome. No, need to thank me; simply sending on your bank details will suffice.

So, if you are sitting comfortably (on the toilet preferably), then I'll begin.

1

INTRODUCTION

THE NIGHTMARE BEFORE CROHN'S

Tuesday 10 August 2010
'…another day of toilet troubles…'

Thursday 19 August 2010
'Another night of agonising pain, didn't sleep a wink, when I tried to get out of bed it was so unbearable I passed out.'

Monday 30 August 2010
'…in pain from the minute I opened my eyes…'

'MY REAR IS IN UPROAR…'

These five little words were one of the first, and most memorable, statements I had written in my diary when I began to realise there was something seriously not quite right 'down there'.

Reading that simple phrase now reminds me quite vividly of the confusion, anger and downright depression

I felt at the time. Pre-diagnosis time, that is. The above statement in itself was surprisingly prudish, despite it having been scrawled in my own personal diary. No one was ever going to see it so why write it in such a cryptic manner? Why not go hell for leather and describe exactly what horrors my 'rear' was experiencing?

After all, the owner of the aforementioned rear would be the only one having the displeasure of reading it.

I can only deduce this enigmatic choice of wording was mainly because I was both embarrassed and ashamed. I was utterly mortified by my gut-churning symptoms and frankly disgusted about what was happening to my own body. That doesn't make it right, or healthy for that matter, but that's exactly how I felt back then. I didn't have the first clue what in the name of David Bowie was happening to me and I was so completely terrified I suppose couldn't even admit those feelings to myself.

Prior to this, using coded or cryptic language in my diary due to embarrassment had only happened once in my recorded history, so far as I can remember anyway. It was when I was of school age, a mere slip of a girl, writing in reference to a crush I had on a boy so much the polar opposite of me that I couldn't even bear to confess my love to the page. Those records have now been destroyed. As has his reputation no doubt.

But I digress.

So, before we delve too deeply into my own personal intestinal tale, let's go right back to basics for the uninitiated. *What exactly IS Crohn's Disease?*

Allow me to put you out of your misery. Crohn's is a form of Inflammatory Bowel Disease known as a 'chronic inflammatory disease', which can affect any part of the gastrointestinal tract (the digestive system) from the patient's purdy mouth to their not-so-purdy anus. Its worst effects are generally based around the colon and ileum.

For the anatomically challenged, the ileum is the final section, or 'end', of the small intestine. This bad boy is about four metres long and extends from the middle section of the small intestine to what's called the 'ileocecal valve', which empties into the colon, or large intestine. The ileum is specifically responsible for the absorption of vitamin B12 and bile salts, amongst other decidedly more unsavoury things. Much like many other parts of the human anatomy, it doesn't *look* too attractive but it is a very important piece of equipment. Thankfully this one is internal.

Crohn's Disease provides its inheritors with some staggeringly gut-churning symptoms. Most common of these are (often excruciating) abdominal pain, severe diarrhoea, uncontrollable bowel movements, weight loss, malnourishment, bleeding from the under carriage... need I go on?

Ok, if you insist...swelling of the stomach, ulcers, lesions, anaemia, arthritis, joint pain...

Although the symptoms are normally most severe around the colon and intestines, Crohn's tends to take itself on a whistle-stop tour of the human body. It also affects several areas of the outside casing as well as pummelling the inside. Let me attempt to explain:

The Crohn's Tour stops off at the skin, making it dry, irritated and painful, breaking it out and leaving you in the unfortunate position where the mirror starts to become your mortal enemy and it feels as though a paper bag on the head would be a preferable look.

We then head towards the head and more precisely the scalp, again leaving the patient in a state of mild torture, where even brushing your hair can hurt as it falls out in clumps. In my case, I quickly became accustomed to removing wig-worthy amounts of my own hair from the shower drain every morning. In the long term I've found, much to my dismay, that the condition has also left my hair in terrible condition: limp, lifeless and with split ends who are never, ever getting back together.

Crohn's then travels further on to the rest of your limbs, making your bones and body ache and leaving you feeling wrung out like a wet rag, and with decidedly less spark than a defunct 40-year-old generator.

In the history books (being as vague, as is my wont, here), the cause of Crohn's Disease is officially recorded as: 'environmental, immunological and bacterial factors', resulting in 'chronic inflammatory disorder', whereby the body's immune system attacks the digestive system. This basically means our bodies are fighting against us thereby, doing the polar opposite of what we want and *need* them to.

As yet, doctors and scientists, and other similarly brainy people, still don't know exactly what causes the disease or why it affects such a wide and varied range of people. It's commonly known that the illness initially tends to present symptoms in the patients' twenties and thirties, with another peak in their fifties and seventies. But Crohn's can really occur at any age. It is currently most prevalent in 25–30-year-olds.

The disease is not hereditary; however, there is unfortunately a genetic link with Crohn's Disease whereby siblings of affected patients can find themselves at a higher risk of developing the condition. This was something both my brothers were understandably concerned about when I finally had my official diagnosis.

As yet there is no known cure for the condition, either pharmaceutical or surgical. Treatment options for Crohn's are sorely limited to controlling the symptoms, maintaining or prolonging periods of remission and preventing relapses. It's widely known that smoking affects Crohn's patients much more than those who don't partake in a wee puff and that it can serve to exacerbate existing symptoms. Current statistics confirm that smokers are twice as likely to develop Crohn's as non-smokers.

Quick potted history: Crohn's Disease took its name from the doctor who first discovered the condition way back in 1932. Together with two of his then colleagues, the gastroenterologist Burrill Bernard Crohn (see what he did there?) described a series of patients at Mount Sinai Hospital in New York with 'inflammation of the terminal ileum', the area most commonly affected by the illness.

However, many years prior to this initial discovery, in 1904, 'ileitis terminalis' was first described by the Polish surgeon Antoni Leśniowski. Regardless, due to the precedence of Crohn's name in the alphabet, it later became known in worldwide literature as Crohn's Disease. Only in Poland does it continue to be named Leśniowski-Crohn's Disease. Poor chap, something as simple as the alphabet standing in the way of his claim to medical fame. I suppose it's a blessing to all patients like me that Crohn's surname was not something more obvious like Winterbottom or Smellie...

But I think that's probably more than enough of the facts and figures, which is a great relief for me as that was pretty much the sum of all I know about the origin of the disease.

What I'm personally more concerned with now is the future. My future, that of my fellow patients and how this disease affects and will continue to affect my loved ones.

If we were to look at it in a comic-book-movie style, my Crohn's 'origin story' only started officially in 2009.

THE CHRONIC BOOM

When I take the time to think back to my earlier life all those years back, 'P.C.' (Pre Crohn's), I feel a strange sense of sadness for my former self. In reading my diaries from around that time it's akin to watching a bad film you'd forgotten you were the star of...

I can remember only particular moments, like seemingly endless time spent in hospital becoming obsessed with completing moronic word searches and solely living off painkillers and diluted juice. I *know* a lot of this time I felt low and alone, and was in an almost constant state of worry, always just a blood test away from an anxiety attack.

It's still a bit of a shocker to read just how much pain I was *physically* in and the full extent of my symptoms. Not to mention my mental state. It genuinely feels as if I'm peeking into someone else's medical records. Albeit, slightly more legible ones. Without glittery cat stickers.

This exercise of looking back into the deepest depths of my sickly inner psyche has, however, and thankfully, helped to remind me how far I've come since then. In body and in mind.

The first proper inkling I had there was something very badly wrong with my insides was when I began to experience sharp and surprisingly nasty pains in my stomach. This was a pain all of its own and like nothing I'd ever felt before. I had absolutely no frame of reference for these feelings because this was completely uncharted territory for me. It began like trapped wind – initially mildly painful and irritating and then grew increasingly fierce as the days and weeks went by. The pain became more severe and the periods of discomfort increasingly prolonged and intense. By the time I was eventually hospitalised it was unbearable and I was unable to stand upright.

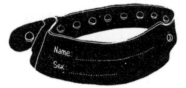

I had felt vaguely similar pain before, but usually only for a few moments and certainly not anywhere near horrific enough for me to complain about (outside of my own head anyway). In my youth I'd probably discounted a lot of this discomfort and these strange feelings as being brought on by period pains or that old chestnut, 'growing pains'. By this point though, I was in my mid-twenties. Growing pains were a thing of the past, and period pain certainly paled in comparison to feeling as though I was suffering contractions 24 hours a day.

Perhaps surprisingly, knowing what I do now, I didn't worry too much about this consistent aching at the time. I suppose I had banked on the pain lasting no more than a few days and eventually subsiding of its own accord; although it's crystal clear to see now that this had no intention of ever happening.

I became more and more frustrated at my own body. I tried to cut some things out of my diet that my parents and I thought might be upsetting me. I started to drink less caffeine, cut out fizzy drinks and eat more fruit and vegetables, etc.

I was completely unaware that this was all futile and that the disease I was silently suffering from was spreading and becoming decidedly more severe. I was also completely unaware the disease I had even existed.

If this were a straight-to-DVD film, or a bad soap opera, there would be a 'DUM DUM DUUUUM!' right about now. But this is a book, so you'll just have to make that noise in your own heads as you read. (Do I have to do all the work around here?)

Having knowledge of the background of the disease or not, being diagnosed with an incurable illness can be an excruciatingly terrifying time. For me, it was a mixture of several emotions, the most prominent of these being relief. A massive weight was lifted from my shoulders when I finally knew what was wrong with me.

This was closely followed by fear and trepidation. I had absolutely no idea what was ahead of me and if there was any potential solution.

Strangely, I also felt a huge sense of validation. It was finally being confirmed at long last that the pain I was feeling was not just in my head. I wasn't a massive hypochondriac with zero tolerance for pain. It was real, and there was a reason for it.

For many new patients, and perhaps even families and friends of patients, these feelings I have described will most likely strike a chord. Many new 'Crohnies' (still not sure how I feel about giving us a 'name' like some sort of diseased gang none of us chose to become members of) find it difficult to understand the full complexities of the disease, especially if their doctors are not particularly blessed in the art of explaining the condition in layman's terms. It's difficult news to grasp at any time of life, but for young people possibly even harder to get to grips with. They may be too young to fully understand what lies ahead, which I suppose can be both a curse and a blessing.

It can take a long time to come to terms with, and you may feel, at first, almost as though you are grieving. When you are first told you have an incurable illness, it is natural to progress through the stages of grief. Denial, then self-inflicted isolation, anger, depression... It can be especially hard to digest (pun always intended) if you don't know anyone with the condition or don't have knowledge of it yourself. It can often be a very lonely and distressing time.

To this day, I often feel this apparent grief for my former life. This feeling comes in spurts and normally goes just as quickly as it comes. Much like a continually disappointing lover, one may say.

Like any loss in life it's something you rarely 'get over', you just gradually learn to live without it. The trouble with this particular loss is that as patients we *are* still living with it. Grieving is commonly a very slow and painful process, especially when you find yourself fighting the murderer of your former life on a daily basis. A slightly disturbing analogy perhaps, but a lot of sick leave makes for a lot of crime-drama viewing. In fact, my bathroom has looked not unlike a grisly scene from CSI many a time.

In my case, I was eventually diagnosed at 27 years old, yet it was the first time I'd even so much as heard the name of the condition, let alone known what it entailed. Again, unfortunately, this is not uncommon. Most patients find themselves in the position where they are suddenly saddled with an illness they don't know the first thing about. It's frightening yet reassuring to know that what you are going through is a genuine condition. With a real name and everything!

When the initial shock of understanding that Crohn's is incurable passes (as much as it can at that point), the focus then turns to what can be done to get the immediate symptoms under control. Which is certainly easier said than done…

CROHN OF CONTENTION

The first major clue I was suffering with Crohn's Disease was when I was diagnosed with arthritis at the supposedly sprightly age of 25 years old. Arthritis is a condition widely associated with Crohn's Disease.

It can also be a major clue in the diagnosing of Crohn's. In finally becoming aware of this link, and in trying to get to the bottom of my own mystery illness, I began to feel somewhat cunning and intuitive, much like that enigmatic TV detective, Columbo.

Although without the mac, cigar, ability to notice a major clue or penis.

I had been experiencing some sharp pain in one of my knees for a good few months before finally taking the plunge and hobbling up the hill to visit the doctor. Initially I was told I had probably just sprained my leg and was advised to put frozen peas on it... This was both incredibly humiliating and embarrassing and I felt as if I must've been completely overreacting.

But that's the problem with pain; only *you* know how it feels. Only *you* know your own body and only *you* know that something is seriously out of the ordinary. It can, at times, be incredibly hard to convey these feelings to others. But a little more on that later...

Eventually, after trying (and promptly discarding) the pea-related advice, the swelling and the pain developed and became so insufferably brutal that it was increasingly difficult to walk, let alone dance all night to David Bowie and bad 1980s power ballads. I tottered back to the surgery and persuaded them to, at the very least, grant me an X-ray. Peas be with you.

Shortly after this was performed, I was diagnosed with arthritis. Since then, I've had cortisone injections, heavy-duty painkillers and bouts of physiotherapy. Unfortunately, nothing seemed to put a dent in the pain. I had no clue at this point of course that this particular pain would soon be the least of my worries...

My own Crohn's diagnosis was an incredibly trying and lengthy process. This isn't entirely unusual; in fact, it's mainly to be expected, as the disease itself can be so irritatingly difficult to pinpoint.

After stumbling back and forth from my doctors' surgery in agony for several months, and with seemingly no progress or chance of any form of resolution in sight, I was feeling almost unbearably frustrated and disheartened. The GP's initial suggestions at my complaints of intense stomach pain varied from the insulting to the ridiculous. Keeping it short, as I have only several pages to work with, these included: my diet, trapped wind, period pain and growing pains (I was 26 at this point). As I had minimal medical knowledge and no alternative, I attempted to change my diet to suit these potential diagnoses: eat more fruit, less green veg and more green veg, cut out fizzy drinks and drink more water – all to no avail. It really didn't matter one iota what I ate or drank, the pain was relentless and almost instantaneous when swallowing so much as a morsel of food. In fact, it became increasingly obvious that the cause of this misery seemed to be directly linked to my taking in of food and drink. As the pain increased and my appetite all but curled up and died, I swiftly began to feel irritable and hopeless and started to wonder whether or not the pain *was* all in my head after all. I was snapping at everyone, I was eating less and I was barely sleeping. I felt as if I was going slowly mad. *I knew* I felt this pain, yet I seemed to be completely incapable of convincing anyone else to believe me.

My first sniff of progress eventually came when, after visiting my GP for what seemed like the 45 millionth time in breathtakingly crippling pain, I was initially diagnosed with suspected appendicitis. The doctor couldn't be sure and as she was thankfully reluctant to take any chance of things escalating (or, I'd imagine, the surgery getting sued), I was promptly rushed to hospital on the assumption I'd be having my appendix removed.

This regrettably transpired not to be the case, and after being discharged with enough pain relief to flatten an elephant, it wasn't too long before I was back in hospital with these same mysterious symptoms again. And then again. And *again*… Repeat to fade.

I distinctly remember desperately wishing that it *had* been appendicitis I'd been dealing with – at least that way I would have been post-op and in the stages of recovery by now. The pain that was currently ruling my life would have been in a surgical waste disposal somewhere and I'd be looking forward to a symptom-free future. Instead, I was *still* suffering and seemingly still no further forward. In fact, I felt that I'd taken 12 wobbly steps back.

During these countless trips to the doctors and stays in hospital, I was attempting as best I could to carry on my 'normal' life around my 'sick' one. I was working full time and trying to eat as well as maintain some semblance of a social life. These activities were NOT easy in the slightest. The simplest of tasks had suddenly become gargantuan feats of human strength that I simply did not possess.

One of my lowest points pre-diagnosis came when I was walking to work one morning.

By now I was accustomed to being awoken at around 4.00 am each day by agonising stomach cramps and having to spend the next few hours half asleep on the toilet. This had just become part of my routine. I obviously wasn't happy about it but by this point I'd almost accepted this pain as being my life and just got on with it. As you can, no doubt, imagine I was consistently shattered and my whole body ached to extremes.

Under normal circumstances, my walk to work takes around 10–15 minutes. This particular morning in question it took me over an HOUR. I almost passed out several times and tried with all my might (not that I had much might…) to focus on the building I was desperately wobbling towards. It was like my personal Mecca. All I could think about was getting there. If I could just get there I'd be alright. I'd be able to sit down, go to the toilet, throw up. I'd be alright. Focus. One foot in front of the other. Focus. Focus.

When I eventually made it to my desk, I fell into my chair. A colleague saw my ashen face and the sight of me clutching my stomach and asked 'Are you ok? '

That was it. Like a bolt from the blue, those three words were all I needed to hear. I collapsed into tears and mumbled something along the lines of, 'No, I'm really not. I think I need to go to the hospital.' In that moment I'd finally accepted I couldn't cope with this on my own any more and that rather than being 'ok' I was truly the polar opposite. I needed help in dealing with the pain and in getting to the bottom of what was causing it. I desperately craved someone qualified to listen and understand that this agony was not merely in my head. Up to this point I think I'd felt that because I'd complained about this discomfort for so long and couldn't 'prove' it, I'd soon start to push away the people closest to me when they inevitably began to doubt my relentless protestations of pain. I'd felt trapped and angry at anyone glancing at me with as much as a glimmer of doubt in their eyes. I didn't want to be alone with my pain anymore.

Most importantly, I needed to be completely honest and explain exactly what was happening to my body.

I went to hospital again that morning and when I came out, this time a few weeks later, I was awaiting tests to confirm the suspected diagnosis of Crohn's Disease.

I was all at once confused, relieved and validated. Not to mention utterly and completely terrified.

INTO THE DANGER CROHN

Without intending to compound any potential fears, diagnosis can be an incredibly scary time – for everyone concerned, not just the patient. You may initially feel bathed in relief at knowing what you are dealing with, but that bliss is usually swiftly replaced with gut-wrenching fear and trepidation at what lies ahead. You can be left feeling lost and clueless. You may feel you are drifting on a bit of a downward spiral, which is completely understandable.

So what tips can I, as a fairly seasoned Crohn's sufferer myself, offer in dealing with the big, bad, scary diagnosis?

1. CROHN IN 60 SECONDS

Don't panic. This is much, much easier said than done. Believe me, I know.

All you can hear right now are the words 'incurable', 'disease', 'chronic' *et al.* and you are thinking only the worst. It's all understandably terrifying. Try, if you can, not to pick out and focus too much on these singular 'shock' words or phrases, and listen very carefully and intently to what the doctor is telling you. Don't typically assume the worst (whatever the 'worst' is for you) before knowing all the facts. It's a lot to take in, so don't pressure yourself into accepting your situation overnight. Think positively wherever possible! Remember, at the very least, now that you know what's wrong, you have something to research. So get studying!

2. SHERLOCK CROHN'S

Learn all you can about your new condition.

Soak up all the information the doctor/consultant/ surgeon/nurse can give you and ask him or her ANYTHING and everything you are unsure of. There is no such thing as a stupid question where the unknown is concerned so, whatever you do, don't allow yourself to feel ashamed of quizzing the health professionals while you have the chance. All of this is happening to YOU – they will understand your natural concern and anxiety.

The internet is also a wonderful learning tool, but try initially to stick to sites such as blogs or forums created and written by patients for patients. Vague information is invalid information. Hear anything 'medical' direct from someone qualified – either patient or professional.

'Layman's terms' can often make it much easier to understand rather than getting bogged down in medical jargon. Patients often also offer a different perspective on living with the condition.

3. DOG WITH A CROHN

Be relentless.

Explain all your symptoms in as much detail as you can. Don't concern yourself with how the more gruesome aspects of your illness come across to others; it's a cliché but your doctors really have heard it all before. As much as you may think it, you are not unique. Being completely open and honest is the only way the doctors can properly establish what course of treatment to start you on. Diagnosis is one thing but it's also incredibly important you know what's next when you leave the hospital. What medications do I have to take and where will I get them? When is my follow-up appointment? Who can I call if I have a flare-up? What support networks do I have outside the hospital walls? If you are baffled by jargon or medical terms, then ensure you don't leave until you understand exactly what is being said. After all it's your body, and it's you who will be taking this illness home with you.

4. MAKE NO CROHN'S ABOUT IT

Don't allow yourself to get caught up in the drama surrounding your illness.

Your friends and family will panic and worry just like you have, which is totally understandable, but let's face it, not exactly helpful. You can get tangled up in trying to calm *them* down when *you* are the one who is incredibly ill yourself. Concentrate solely on your recovery and, if necessary, direct loved ones to your consultants or nurses for more detailed updates. I spent most of my hospital time trying to explain something to my family that I barely had a grasp on myself – frustrating, irritating and distressing in equal measure. The lack of information was upsetting for them, which made me feel I was failing in giving them the outcome they wanted. It's also important to bear in mind the difference between patient and visitor: the Patient wants to see a friendly face, maybe get a cuddle or two, hear your tales from the outside world and mainly get a distraction from their current situation; the Visitor wants to know how you are and when you will get home, what's happening with your recovery, what are the doctors doing and why, '*Oh why* is everything taking *so long*?' Try to meet a happy medium somewhere in the middle.

5. CROHNED TO PERFECTION

If it's a viable option, try to enlist a family member or partner to take care of things for you on the outside of the hospital walls.

Knowing you will be potentially cooped up in hospital for a period of time can be incredibly stressful, especially if you have responsibilities at home that won't wait for you to recover. Handing over the task of things such as dealing with bills, looking after pets and the safety of your home can be a huge weight lifted off your shoulders, allowing you to focus on getting well again.

Giving someone at your work a contact instead of always having to deal with them yourself can also be a relief and take some of the panic away from speaking to a potentially irritable and stressed employer. This caused me no end of worry – my boss at the time was pressuring me for a return date when I didn't have the first clue when I'd get home, let alone back to work. Stalking the wards with a drip dragging behind you trying to get a phone signal to apologise for lack of attendance is really not what you need when you are already unfeasibly ill.

Although the world won't stop turning simply because you are medically incarcerated, you have to try to put all of the little energy you do have into getting better.

6. CROHNLY THE BRAVE

Chin up and calm down.

You are ill and will now most likely be ill for a long time to come. But you will also leave the hospital feeling *better*. Much better than you were when you came in anyway, and fingers crossed more hopeful for the months and years to come. You will be taken care of now and be safe in the knowledge that your pain is not being ignored any more. Remember, where possible, to keep track of hospital contacts and names of the consultants/doctors you deal with who know you and your condition well. Having that sort of 'safety net' can be a huge boost. Try to think of a resolution and a comfortable future. Don't go backwards, because putting it bluntly, you have no alternative.

7. HEARD IT THROUGH THE INTESTINE

Ignore scare tactics.

Some, shall we say, *insensitive* people may choose to fill your head with horror stories about your new condition. This may be done by using either (alleged) personal experiences or those of others that they've perhaps heard in passing. Try as best you can to focus on YOU and not be drawn into others' tales of woe.

Remember that everyone has their own reason for telling a story.

When I was diagnosed, I was helpfully told by some lovely people that I would 'go blind', 'have a colostomy bag forever', 'eat through a drip' and 'be on a ventilator'. Or (my personal favourite), simply, 'die'.

These golden nuggets of 'information', as you can imagine, don't help to ease a worried and freshly diseased mind. Some people just don't have that filter in their brain that stops them from saying stupid things. Be as tolerant as you can (after you've beaten them to within an inch of their life, obviously!) and as kindly as you can, advise them you really appreciate their input but you'll probably stick to a medical opinion.

8. A MIND OF MY CROHN

Don't judge your own illness on what you know of others.

If you already have a family member, friend or acquaintance with Crohn's Disease, don't assume that your experiences will be the same. Crohn's patients do share symptoms in common, but each person has unique and individual ways of dealing with them, and each case is always very different. Some patients have incredibly severe cases of the condition whereas others may, thankfully, lead a perfectly 'normal' and healthy life with only a symptom or two rearing its diseased head occasionally. Many find themselves having to become reliant on medication to cope with their illness, while others can find that their Crohn's can be controlled purely by adapting their diet. Although, sadly, these latter cases are much rarer than we would like.

Comparing yourself to others with the same condition can often be a fruitless and time-wasting exercise, as essentially you will feel what your body wants YOU to feel, regardless of what anyone else happens to say or have.

9. THE TWILIGHT CROHN

Push yourself outside your comfort zone.

If you find it too much of a struggle or just downright embarrassing to talk to doctors, don't be afraid to share, in confidence, your more personal problems with people who care for you. The majority of your friends and family will not wince at the mere mention of your backside as much as you may think. Their reactions may pleasantly surprise you and will I hope help give you the confidence to open up to the medical professionals. The more you talk about it the easier it will become.

10. HEART OF CROHN

Don't force yourself to enter a world you aren't ready for.

Many new patients find they are gently encouraged into discussing their condition with other sufferers or joining forums and groups, which they perhaps aren't entirely comfortable with. If that's not for you then steer clear, at the very least until you feel a lot more relaxed in yourself. You absolutely shouldn't feel pressured into anything other than getting well.

However don't rule out these support mechanisms entirely. Certainly don't push yourself to get involved in something you aren't ready for, but don't assume the way you feel now won't change. No one will judge you. No one will feel you are insulting them or that any of your opinions or 'gut feelings' (*PUN CLAXON*) are invalid, because as patients we have all felt them too. If that's any form of comfort for you then reach out and simply ask for the support you need. It can be an invaluable learning tool if nothing else.

HOW FAR CROHN ARE YOU?

It's widely known that very few people are 100 per cent comfortable in discussing their bowel movements, and until I was diagnosed with Crohn's Disease, I would certainly not have considered myself amongst them. It just wasn't really the 'done thing' in my household.

I'm not sure if this mild prudishness goes back generations or was just more of a trait within my own immediate family, but it's certainly something I became more acutely aware of as my problems in that department began to escalate. I realised I felt vaguely uncomfortable and borderline ashamed about discussing anything untoward that may have been happening below the love handles.

I don't, in any way, blame my parents for this. I don't blame anyone, for that matter. It may have absolutely nothing to do with my upbringing, but there was obviously some reason I felt so unpleasant about discussing my own rear end. It's just one of those things I can't quite place.

This 'thing' however, made it decidedly more difficult for me to be as honest as I could with doctors and nurses when they were struggling to diagnose my illness. I felt it was easier to nod in agreement with their suggestions than to express the full extent of the aforementioned 'uproar' I was experiencing down there. I wanted to save myself the red-faced humiliation, and no matter how much I was told they'd 'heard it all before' I couldn't escape the fact that I was actually being forced to talk about POO.

MY poo for that matter.

This fool couldn't handle her own stool.

This missus couldn't discuss her faeces.

This burd couldn't debate her own tur...you get the general idea.

In Crohn's Disease a patient's toilet activities are very important indeed. What ends up in the porcelain can be an incredibly vital clue for doctors in establishing the extent of the disease and its effects on the body. Medical professionals can discover so much from just a small, unassuming stool sample. Not only that, but they can also garner a huge amount of information from simple questioning. All of which means as a patient you really have to get to grips with 'talking shit'. Normally an absolute BLESSING for me.

They will need to know specifics. What consistency is it?

Is there blood in it? How much is there, and how often are you going?

I'm never particularly comfortable with this kind of bizarre quizzing, but I'm slowly trying to learn to get descriptive about it. In fact I now find that more people around me feel they can openly discuss their *own* bowel movements, whether I want to hear about it or not. As though I've unwittingly become some strange form of poo guru. A Poo-ru, if you will. People have started asking me what it means when this, that or the next thing happens in their bathroom. I absolutely do not profess to be any kind of expert on matters of the rear, however I do have extensive knowledge of various unsavoury scenarios that people tend to think gives me insight others perhaps don't possess.

Many new (and old) patients also find this type of 'in-depth' colon-versation difficult to take to at first. Most of these patients, thankfully, find that they eventually become immune to the discussions with medical professionals that take place around that area. They come to realise, as I've had to, that it's essential, unfortunately, in helping the doctors do their job to the best of their abilities. At the end of the day, it's *our* health on the line; therefore we should do everything in our power to help ourselves get better.

I often find myself getting incredibly frustrated by the fact that there still seems to be such a stigma attached to

Crohn's Disease. This stigma spreads itself across several other bowel-related illnesses for that matter.

We, as humans, are all essentially the same; we all take in food and water in the same way and all expel it in the same way too. So why should we be embarrassed to discuss these things openly?

That's not entirely true of course, humans with Crohn's often find their bodies (and in particular their bowels) don't work in quite the same way as those without, however much we would like them too.

When you have been established as a Crohn's patient, you may find a lot of your doctor's time can be spent at your rear end. Not a thought I'm sure you, or your doctor, will particularly relish.

Colonoscopies and other similar procedures can be invasive and often require 'probing'. You know – that thing that aliens always do in films when they come down to Earth for a visit.

One could certainly say it *is* an alien concept, for a stranger to drug you then shove a camera up your back passage without so much as a mojito for your trouble. *Then*, as if that weren't enough, for you all to sit around and watch the show on a screen! WITHOUT any popcorn. It's an absolute scandal! I exaggerate, obviously; you do get a mojito (if you go private).

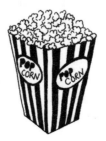

As I recall, my first of my many colonoscopies was not a particularly pleasant experience. Although I would say it never really is for anyone (sadists aside perhaps).

When the time for a scope approaches, in order to make the experience somewhat more bearable, I like to think of the whole procedure as a series of steps. This makes it much easier for me to focus on the end result. I do this in much the same way that I got through the trial of attending Catholic Mass in my youth. Simply by slowly reading through my wee Mass book along with the priest as he worked his magic on the crowd, awaiting the final hymn with glee, knowing that in less than ten minutes I'd be home free! Free to spend the rest of my Sunday eating steak pie and watching the omnibus of Sunset Beach.

So, with my master plan in mind, here are my tried and tested 'Colonosco-Steps'.

Try saying that after a few vodkas. Or after a colonoscopy for that matter...

The 24 hours prior to your procedure will be spent 'prepping' your bowels for the big event. It's essential your insides are completely empty (or as close as you can get) before the procedure. This will ensure the doctor gets the best view of what's going on inside. This unfortunately requires fasting and drinking nothing but water and what will seem like gallons of fluid. Alongside this H2O you'll swill a horrible drink that will normally be 'lemon flavour' or something equally as rancid (like no lemon I've ever found on planet Earth – again, an alien concept).

Then you are required to panic mildly and probably whine about nothing happening 'down there' for a while, awaiting the floodgates opening. This is followed VERY closely by spending the rest of your day rushing back and forward in desperation to the toilet until you are left with nothing but skin, bones, a sore backside and a horrible lemonesque taste in your mouth.

The procedure itself can be done with or without anaesthetic (I personally always opt for the drugs) and is a pretty quick process. You are asked to relax as much as you are able and are then given a mild sedative whilst the doctors take over and a camera (almost as small as a matchstick) is inserted into your back passage. This is skilfully manoeuvred around your intestines until a good picture of the affected area(s) is found. Usually biopsies are taken for testing. You can opt to remain awake throughout the event and watch the inside of your body in 3D or allow yourself to drift into la-la land and preferably wake up when it's all over. My first colonoscopy was a very stressful experience, as I was completely uptight about what lay ahead. Second time round I knew exactly what to expect so I allowed myself to try to remain as calm and relaxed as I could. I knew this time that tensing up wouldn't help me, or the doctor, one iota.

This last one does vary on where in the world this procedure is performed, but in the UK when the scope is over you are blessed with the chance of a brief snooze until you are fully back in reality and a sandwich at the end of it for your trouble. In various other parts of the globe doctors may prefer the patient to introduce foods again slowly, starting with something easily digestible like soup. That's unfortunate, as the sandwich is my absolute *favourite* bit. I devour that bread and ham double as if I've just been stranded on a desert island for three months. Or sat through every series of Lost from start to finish. Whichever feels longest.

COLON, I'M COMIN'

Whatever your length of experience with Crohn's Disease, it's generally accepted that colonoscopies, endoscopies and similar procedures are rarely delighted in. They are, by and large, unpleasant and uncomfortable yet, unfortunately, essential. They are one of the best and most accurate ways in which to establish the extent of symptoms and serve as a wonderful diagnostic tool. It was only following my first scope that it was confirmed I had the condition, and then the treatment could finally begin. That was a happy day.

It's exceptionally important not to fear the methods health professionals may have to use to help you. At the root of it, that's all they are trying to do. If you feel afraid and anxious about any aspects of your diseased journey it is imperative you speak up about it. Doctors and nurses are there to help make the whole process as easy as possible for you, but they can only do that when they know the full story.

Crohn's is scary, and everything that will inevitably get inserted into your every nook and cranny may be even scarier, but those are the moments in which you need to open up (potentially in more ways than one…).

Reaching out your hand to ask for help is one of the most intimidating things you can do, and I've personally struggled to accept that I need those hands over the last few years. If you ever ask me how I am I will pretty much

ALWAYS relay that old chestnut, 'I'm fine'. It drives people around me crazy. I'm never, or at least rarely ever, fine. It's just 100 per cent easier than constantly complaining or having to relay the same old story. No one who loves me wants me to feel anything less than fine and I don't want them to be forced to share my pain.

A similar scenario rears its head in the doctor's surgery. I don't want them to think of me as a hypochondriac, yet I want them to be blessed with some sixth sense that allows them to treat me without all the facts. It's an impossible expectation, and highly illogical, Captain.

In all seriousness, anyone who is having a hard time dealing with their illness and all it entails may need someone to talk to from time to time. Even if that person can't help, it's often a massive boost in itself just conversing outside of your own head about how you are feeling. I know that my partner, friends and family can't cure my disease. But I also *know* they would love to, and often simply hearing that is enough. I recognise that when I feel a little better I can laugh heartily at the times when I felt utterly pathetic. Like those Saturday nights when I occasionally weep into my cat's fur solidly for prolonged periods whilst eating Nutella from the jar and listening to 'Crying' by Roy Orbison.

It's disheartening to know that these 'moments' will happen again and again, but also a little reassuring. I don't ever want to pretend this part of my life doesn't exist and I don't ever want to feel alone. No one should ever have to. I have to suffer from this disease but it also affects everyone I love, so why shouldn't I let them share in the good *and* the bad with me?

If you are afraid of something as small as a tiny camera being wiggled about your colon, to something as massive as living with a life-changing illness, talk to someone about how low you feel when you need to. Let them help. In my experience, someone around you will always want to.

2

ADAPTING

THE CROHN RANGER

Saturday 28 August 2010
'No energy, no motivation to do anything today, at a loss as to what's happening to me and how to get out of this hole.'

Thursday 2 September 2010
'He woke me up coming in, I was so tired and in so much pain I couldn't stop crying. Pathetic. He said he understands but when he asks what he can do I am reluctant to reply because I'm so frustrated at the knowledge there's nothing he can do and that's not his fault.'

ATTACK OF THE CROHN'S

Now, perhaps you are reading my little diseased story so far and thinking, 'Jeez, what an absolute *drama queen!*'

Perhaps you have been quite seriously ill yourself and feel my particular responses to my condition were typically 'girly' and perhaps even potentially embarrassing overreactions.

So, to you doubting Thomases or Thomasinas, let me (as calmly as I can) ask you this: have you ever in your life been so frustrated you think you may explode?

(Please stop giggling at the back.)

Have you ever felt that no relief will ever come?

(Seriously, grow up.)

Or that as things have become so bad you will have to take matters entirely into your own hands?

(Right, that's ENOUGH, DETENTION!)

It's a horribly slippery slope that leads from persistent pain towards depression. Those who have, thankfully, never had to experience the level of pain Crohn's can reach can't begin to understand how it feels to live your life in that way. In what can only be described as constant agony and gut-crunching misery. That first part was a lie actually. There are many other ways it can be described, but those mostly contain profanities and my mum might read this so I'm not going down that road.

When you've popped a million pills (doctor-prescribed pills that is, and not all at once obviously, kids), you've tried everything the doctors suggest however fruitless you KNOW it may be, your body is ravaged, you are limp and feel the life draining from you and yet, at the end of it all, after going through test after test, tubes attached to every available orifice, body left like a pin cushion and enough blood drained from you to fill a swimming pool, you find you are STILL IN PAIN.

For me, after trying countless treatments, a variety of different drugs and relentless changes to my diet, the final option was to refer me for surgery. A 'resection', to give the procedure I underwent its official medical name. Without getting into the nitty-gritty too much, this type of operation requires removal of part or all of the diseased area, usually concerning the bowel and/or intestines. For me, they removed a particularly foul part of my insides on my left hand side, so mean and nasty it apparently would have attempted to kill me had it been left to its own devices for much longer. What an absolute bastard.

However, before my guts were to be introduced to a shiny scalpel, I first had to endure a meet and greet with my potential surgeon…

My first consultation with him did not go well, to put it mildly. He was decidedly unimpressed by having to spend any time with me and from the get-go his attitude stunk to high heaven. Now, before I go any further, bear in mind that when meeting with this man I was in no means, by this point, of sound mind. I was in crippling and consistently agonising pain for which there was seemingly no relief. I was blinded by relentless pain and misery. I was mentally and physically a complete wreck, badly anaemic, light as a feather, utterly hopeless and mentally drained and this meeting appeared to me as a massive light at the end of an incredibly dark and diseased tunnel.

I'd been led to believe this meeting was pretty much a formality and I'd wrongly assumed that after talking to him he would see me for the absolute shell of a woman I'd become – void of mental and physical strength. He'd hear just how bad things really were and fit me in for a slicin' ASAP! I now know just how unbearably naïve of me that was.

(I should also make a point of mentioning that this was only my personal experience and not a sweeping generalisation on surgeons in general. I think they are beyond wonderful at what they do.)

So, instead of the Disney-style outcome I'd imagined whereby I hugged the surgeon with tears in my eyes and a troop of nurses waltzed in to carry me to the operating theatre on a gurney singing 'Dr Feelgood', what actually happened was disappointingly different. The man in question couldn't be bothered to look at my notes, let alone come at me with a scalpel or a twee cuddle. He got our meeting underway with the sensitive opening gambit of 'Why are you even here?' He then rhymed off a staggering list of treatments (the vast majority of which I'd already tried) and voiced in no uncertain terms (and in his own words, of course) that he would be going nowhere near me with so much as a butter knife until I'd tried all of the aforementioned list. He practically shrugged me out of the office as a waste of his valuable time.

Now don't get me wrong, I am well aware he must be an incredibly busy man. I'm also 99.9 per cent certain I would not have been the only patient he would see that day or perhaps the most unwell of his patients. I am by no means self-absorbed enough not to realise that there are people in situations much worse than my own. But to make another human feel they are unworthy of a few moments of your time when they are laying out their worst fears and feelings of utter hopelessness right before your eyes, to me is just beggars belief.

Before I was impolitely sent on my decidedly un-merry way, Surgeon Extraordinaire took a moment to advise me that I really wouldn't want to get this sort of operation anyway, as there was a 90 per cent chance I'd require either a temporary or permanent colostomy. He kindly reminded me I was: '…a young woman, and what young woman wants to have a BAG?!'

I advised him that I honestly didn't care what the outcome was, as I was just so desperate for the pain to subside (sounding, I'm pretty sure, increasingly like a junkie looking for a fix) and that I was willing to do my utmost to adapt to it. He told me in no uncertain terms how horrid my life would be if I were to have one, and that if I was in any doubt how awful this would be he'd get the stoma nurse to meet with me to explain a few 'home truths', and prove his point.

I left his office in tears. Not a sobbing mess, but crying those dry, angry tears that take about a week to actually fall from your eye because your face is so COMPLETELY TAUT WITH RAGE. I couldn't believe the way he'd so quickly just discounted my every, and genuine, complaint. I felt foolish and immature. I felt completely worthless and like a total hypochondriac. I felt worse than when I'd gone in, and went home to cry huge, pillow-drenching tears until my ducts ran dry.

A few weeks went by and I was to meet with my original consultant to discuss the potential surgery. When I entered her office she was buoyed, hopeful and smiling. She rightly assumed I would be in the same positive mood, until I explained how badly my meeting with the surgeon had gone. She was angrier than I've ever seen a medical professional. Other than in that ER programme with George Clooney, but they're obviously all acting so it doesn't really count.

She explained she would try to deal with the situation quickly, as she knew how utterly broken I was. She swiftly arranged a meeting with the surgical board to plead my case.

It wasn't long before I was back in her office again, and soon I was checking in to hospital to undergo the surgery she was still utterly insistent I needed. I couldn't believe it. By this point, I was so completely shattered by the whole shambles that I still didn't think it would actually happen until I saw a variety of experts in greens wielding scalpels and suchlike.

As promised, my consultant bravely fought my corner. I like to think physically as well as verbally, ending with her 'clotheslining' the horrid surgeon and victoriously throwing him out of the ring, whilst screaming 'KATHLEEEEEN! KATHLEEEEEEEN!'

However, I'm aware I may be confusing real-life with Rocky again.

QUEENS OF THE CROHN AGE

When the time finally came, a wonderful female surgeon performed my operation and it was a resounding success. I awoke from my drug-induced slumber to find the most badly affected area had been completely removed and I was left with a really neat and tidy scar, and no colostomy bag.

Funnily enough, the surgeon who'd initially declined my bowel access to his scalpel spotted me in the ward one afternoon during my recovery. I haven't seen a man exit a room so quickly since my dad walked in on me holding hands with my first boyfriend. I was almost convinced I saw sparks emanating from his shoes. Although it should be noted for the record that I was on a substantial amount of drugs; he could've been wearing clown shoes for all I knew.

After my surgery and on my release from hospital, I was advised to take time off from work for a few months to rest, recover and begin to rebuild my broken body. This was a very long and arduous process. One much more difficult than I'd initially bargained for.

Never having undergone a procedure anywhere near as serious as this before, and having been in such unbearable pain in the 12 months prior to my surgery, I was both anxious in the extreme at the thought of having to adapt to the outcome of life post-surgery, and absolutely desperate to get it over with and attempt to get back to 'normal'. It's quite clear to see there was a bit of a contradiction in terms going on in my psyche at that point. I wanted complete freedom from the pain and to be able to live my life again, just as I had before all this pesky 'being ill' palaver started.

I'm not really sure what exactly I'd thought would happen when I got home and back into life outside the ward. Best-case scenario, I'd be pain free and my bowels would play a beautiful digestive symphony like never before. Worst-case scenario, I'd be in more pain, the op wouldn't have worked and I'd also have a colostomy bag to adapt to.

I suppose I was slightly blind-sighted as to just what this particular operation would do for me. I was acutely aware I would not be cured. The doctors made sure to imprint that on me whenever possible. I wasn't under any illusions my disease would be gone, and I knew all the potential risks ahead. I was mentally prepared for what was to come because I had to be; the alternative of a life in excruciating pain was too much to contemplate.

One of the main 'dangers' in undergoing this type of surgery was being left with a stoma; an opening created surgically, designed in order to divert the flow of faeces and/or urine. I was, in fact, told I would most likely have a colostomy bag for several months, if not the remainder of my life, as a result of my surgery. This is very common with this type of operation.

It seems churlish knowing what I know of colostomies/ostomies now, and the people living with them, but in my mind back then, this certainly was the hardest thing to deal with.

(* WARNING: POO REFERENCE *)

For anyone unaware, a colostomy bag is a small pouch worn on the outside of the body in cases where parts of, or the whole of, the patient's bowel have been removed. It's there to allow faeces to pass through the body directly into the bag rather than exiting by the traditional method of the back passage. It's a bag that patients have to change regularly themselves and can be with the body for anything from a few months at a time to a lifetime. How long the patient lives with the bag can depend on several factors, including the severity of the illness, volume of surgery required and success (or failure) of any operations. Many patients find, in time, that they prefer having the bag. They feel more freedom and control with it and begin to enjoy the aspect of not having to rush to and from the toilet every five minutes. They feel relief at what they see as getting their independence back and there being no risk of incontinence and find they generally experience a reduction in, or even a complete relief from, pain.

It's no overnight success, of course, and no miracle remedy. There still must be allowances made for the bag. For example, certain foods should be avoided. Oh, and, of course, the disease is still incurable, bag or no bag.

For me, at first anyway, I worried incessantly that suddenly having this bag attached to my body would render me unappealing and a drain on my partner. I fretted about how others would take the news and if my friends would be embarrassed of, or for, me. I got myself into a mild panic about how long it would take me to adapt to having this alien 'thing' on the outside of my body and if I would be repulsed at the sight of myself. Vanity crept in and I stressed about my wardrobe and what clothes I'd be able to wear to keep it firmly out of sight. I worried about eating with it. I worried about swimming. I worried about it bursting. I worried about losing intimacy with my partner. I worried about sex. I worried a LOT.

However, all these initial fears were, thankfully, unfounded, and they were massively outweighed by the immense pain I'd been in during this time.

With the help and reassurance of my partner, I managed to get over my anxious nature and most of my concerns. I began to realise that even if I did have this bag, I would be ALIVE, and not living a life of constant pain and misery. I tried to focus on that and push through my fears.

I also felt a twinge of guilt at having doubted my loved ones' abilities to adapt to this change to my life. They had yet to let me down, so why would they suddenly desert me now? My vanity had gotten the better of me and I tarred those around me with the same brush.

I knew having a colostomy bag would be incredibly hard to adapt to, but that the worst of my disease would be gone. I understood it would be a massive change to my lifestyle, initially anyway, at least until I learned to adjust to it. But the worst of the pain (for now at least) would be over. With all this in mind it made it so much easier to walk into that hospital on the morning of my operation.

As did my mum, clinging on to my wobbly hand for dear life. If anything, it was probably harder for her, having to wave me off as I faded into a prep room to slip into something decidedly less comfortable.

As soon as she was out of sight, I suddenly felt almost unbearably alone, and the fear at what was to come started to kick in. Waiting for any procedure in hospital is generally fine as long as you don't think about it. Although this is easier said than done when you are surrounded by fellow sick people rocking surgical stockings, in a room scented with the nasal-tingling aroma of bleach.

While I awaited my name being called like some perverse game of bingo, I distinctly remember a programme about people searching for antiques in their attics being on TV before I was wheeled off for my op. I also recall thinking how wonderful it would be to find a gem in *my* loft; how much of a difference thousands of pounds would make to *my* life. Then instantly shooting that thought down with the simple fact that all the cash in the world wouldn't stop me having to go through this. I burst into tears and only just managed to pull myself together in time for the nurse to come in and put me at ease with friendly chatter and wonderful, wonderful anaesthesia....

As I've mentioned, my surgery was, thankfully, a huge success and I woke up without a colostomy bag but with a big and gorgeously neat scar. The surgeons advised me they had removed the most badly diseased area and that I should start to heal as well as could be expected. It's clear to see now that I did underestimate quite how much pain I'd be in after the operation though. This was an entirely different variety of pain. I had naïvely expected to be relatively 'pain free' (whatever that means), and I was, to a certain extent. Certainly free of Crohn's pain, but now dealing with the intense ache of having had my stomach opened up and a piece of me cut out.

After the surgery I was taken to a high dependency ward where morphine and I quickly became BFFs. The nurses caring for me were quite wonderful, and when the idea of sitting upright for the first time was put to me it was a huge source of amusement. For me and my morphine-fuelled head that is, but not for the nurses. It hurt to do absolutely anything and everything. I couldn't move, sneeze, cough, turn over or even so much as hiccup. The last things you think about pre-op. Basic human functions suddenly become terrifying. When the doctors told me I could get home – once I'd successfully passed wind and then my first stool – it was as though they'd told me to climb Mount Kilimanjaro wearing nothing but slippers.

I was quite happy to be left in the same position on my hospital bed forever, because the alternative seemed too unbearably grim for words.

Obviously I got up, with a *lot* of help. I gradually learned how to walk and shower and dress myself again. A process I absolutely hated whilst being in hospital – the feeling that you have to rely on someone to do such private things as washing your more...intimate areas. I remember, when showering for the first time after my operation, the nurse suggesting we should remove my bandage to allow me to clean and let my wound heal properly. I laughed at her ludicrous idea, then grimaced and braced for the rip of the bandage, all the while stupidly asking her if she was squeamish and apologising profusely for the state of my wounded stomach. Nurse: squeamish? Goodness me, that morphine was lovely wasn't it?

I wouldn't even consider myself to be particularly prudish, and the shame and embarrassment isn't particularly in a stranger seeing my bits and bobs; it's more about the idea of losing your dignity when you already feel so extraordinarily vulnerable. Your dignity is often something I feel you have to leave firmly at the door upon entering a hospital.

JUST THE CROHNIC

Around the start of 2011, as a new year began, for me it seemed like the end rather than a new beginning. I was utterly hopeless and the idea that I would have to go through horrific surgery with the possibility of months of recovery, a colostomy bag and a lifelong scar was almost too much to bear.

As I've mentioned, by the eventual arrival of my operation I was seriously ill. I had, within the six months prior, rapidly gone downhill. I was not eating, because it simply wasn't possible, I was in gut-wrenching agony every day, which no form of pain relief could touch, I couldn't sleep or walk further than a few steps without almost passing out and, most alarmingly, I'd all but given up mentally. Now don't get me wrong here – I was depressed, yes, but I hadn't given up on life. At least I hadn't given up on the lives of others anyway. I was completely in love with my partner and adored those around me to the point of stalker-ism, so there was absolutely no way on Earth I would have considered doing anything to cause them heartbreak or upset. What I mean is that I had reached a quite devastating point of acceptance. I had come to see that nothing would change for me – no medication or treatment had worked, in fact my medical situation had escalated to the point where I couldn't bear getting out of bed in the morning, so I couldn't see any point in complaining about it. This, in my mind, was my unfortunate life now and I simply had no choice but to get used to it.

This all probably sounds very dramatic, and perhaps self-pitying, but it was merely a way of thinking that my body had driven me to. My particular state of mind was mine, and mine alone, and I in no way used my illness as a means to get attention. That suggestion couldn't have been further from my thoughts (which were predominantly PAINPAINPAINPAIN).

This pain was unbearable and frequently reduced me to tears. I felt I had to try to find a way to fit my *life* around my *illness* – get to and from work, hold down my job and maintain some semblance of a social life, all the while trying to hide the fact that I felt that something was slowly but determinedly ripping my insides out.

Everyone knew. I was, and always will be, a hopeless liar.

I gradually came round to the idea that not only was my approaching operation essential, but it may also actually serve to make me feel better. This seemed such an unlikely resolution that I, illogically, chose not to focus on it and instead worried intensely how I would cope with a potential colostomy bag. Or how brutally unattractive I'd be with a massive scar down my front. I really needn't have worried on either front. I didn't end up with a colostomy bag and my scar hasn't put my partner off the idea of jumping my bones on a regular basis, no more than perhaps having my head and limbs removed might (I like to think that wouldn't, either).

I've come to accept my scarring as a part of my body now, much like my long and decidedly repulsive toe that looks like ET's finger. Although it's fair to say my 'toe acceptance' ended up taking somewhere along the lines of 30 years to take place. To be honest I'm still not quite sure I'm there yet.

HIDEOUS toes aside, I merely relay these thoughts primarily to remind myself that giving up never solved anything. I have felt low since this period before surgery, and I'm 99 per cent sure I will again, but accepting those feelings as a fact of life is where I will always fall down. And stay down. I, and anyone else in my similarly diseased boat, must attempt to remember never to give up hope. It may feel that we are fighting a losing battle with our bodies but it's vital we try not to think of Crohn's as a fight. I feel that way I am constantly setting myself up for a fall. Crohn's is an incurable disease – it will always have the upper hand, but as patients we have functioning minds, and (depending on your religious persuasion), souls; if you choose to use them positively they will always win out.

GO YOUR CROHN WAY

I spent almost the entirety of my twenties focused on suffering from Crohn's Disease. Just existing around my illness seemed to suck up all of my time and energy. My days were spent mainly feeling sick and becoming increasingly frustrated at my worthless body. Everything else around just 'being ill' was a bit of a blur.

When I turned 30, rather than carrying out the suicide I'd planned for such an occasion and/or pummelling myself mentally for not having met my imaginary goals by my imaginary deadline, I chose to embrace ageing, diseased or not. I resolved there was no viable option. Plus I'm too squeamish to kill myself.

The truth is, having accepted age ain't nothin' but a number, I'm now no longer worried about my next decade. Or even my future beyond it for that matter. I'm excited. I'm looking *forward* instead of pointlessly looking back with regret. I plan to face the next few years with the anticipation that things will be infinitely better as I leave my twenties behind.

I'm slowly but surely coming to terms with the fact that Crohn's Disease will always play a massive part in my life. I have resigned myself to working on what I can control – how I let it affect my head and my heart. I even devoted a couple of weeks before my 30th birthday to compiling a list of my own nuggets of advice to my fellow sufferers on living with the disease in the event of you requiring it. Almost like I planned it – here are my 30 musings on the matter.

30. Its ok to feel sad from time to time. Crohn's is a horribly intrusive and all-consuming disease, and no one with as much as an ounce of decency would begrudge you a few moments to wallow. Allow yourself a period to grieve for your old body, your old life and perhaps even the plans you've had to scale down due to your health. Don't be hard on yourself for letting go occasionally.

29. Allow yourself to be cared for. If you are lucky enough to have people in your life who love you and want, and are willing, to help you, then please accept it. Grab it with both hands and don't feel guilty about it. Think about how you would feel if the roles were reversed. Don't be a martyr to your illness.

28. Be prepared for the fact that in undertaking this diseased 'journey', you may lose friends and/or acquaintances. Illness isn't often 'fun', therefore, often in their mind, neither are you. Fun in the conventional sense that is; I don't know about you but evacuating your bowels after a bloated

two hours? Am I right?! The fact that these pre-Crohn's buddies are slowly drifting from your life, much like your capacity to speak coherently on morphine, is really no great loss. The people who are there for you in your time of need are there solely because they love you unconditionally; you'll find them through the mist.

27. Make yourself happy. I'm well aware that this is infinitely easier said than done, but do try your best to bring yourself as much joy as is conceivable when you are well. Find what you love and put what spare energy you have left over into it. Don't let your disease stop you from doing ANYTHING.

26. Be patient. Bear in mind that it may well be a long and arduous road establishing what treatment and medication(s) are going to work best for you. Doctors and nurses are doing their absolute utmost to get you well, so don't make it any harder for either of you during that difficult process.

25. On the other side of the coin, speak up. If you feel let down by any aspect of your treatment, then tell someone. If you are anxious about any piece of advice you have been given, or route you have been instructed to take, it's vital you talk to 'Whom It May Concern'. Don't take no for an answer.

24. Learn all you can about your condition. You, and your loved ones, are in the midst of the most challenging time of your life; you need to be as prepared as you can for what lies ahead. Things

are truly never as bad as they may at first seem, and it makes it a million times easier to deal with whatever's thrown at you when you are forearmed.

23. It might sound a tad hypocritical considering you're reading this in a distinctly personal book, but keep some things *private*. The world and its wife do not need (or want) to know about every latest bowel movement.

22. Protect yourself. Keep the things that matter close and don't allow yourself to get caught up in that which won't keep you warm at night. Treasure what's real and what matters above all else.

21. If you find yourself regularly in and out of hospital, it's a good idea to pack a little toilet bag filled with all your essentials. This alleviates the stress of trying to remember everything you'll need in the panic and worry of a hospital stay. It also makes things easier for your loved ones, leaving them the time to organise everything else. It's a nice idea to pop a wee treat in your hospital hand luggage too, a lovely and unexpected surprise when you find you are at your worst. (See my own personal masterclass in hospital packing a little later.)

20. Focus on the future and not what you've left behind. Unless you are a Time Lord, you don't have the ability to change your past, so instead ensure you don't make any mistakes all over again. If you *are* a Time Lord then HIGH FIVE, BECAUSE THAT IS *AWESOME*.

19. Make some more of those mistakes before your time is up.

18. Maintain your dignity. Remember how utterly humiliating parts of this illness can truly be; don't let those moments change how you feel about yourself in the long term. Don't forget you can pick up any dignity you may feel you've lost on the way back out of the doctor's surgery.

17. Try not to allow yourself to be driven to distraction by other people's apparently 'deadly' illnesses – bear in mind that for someone who has never been ill a day in their life, the flu *will* feel as if they are dying. It's easy to become irritated by hypochondriacs; rise above it and don't get drawn into medical discussions. Ill health is not a war. You will most likely trump them every time anyway, perhaps literally if they deserve it.

16. Don't become a health bore.

15. Or a bore.

14. Or an eyesore. Take some pride in how you appear – it can actually serve as a decent tool for dragging yourself from your diseased bed and work as a little pick-me-up.

13. Tell your mum and dad you love them. If you are lucky enough to have them in your life, cherish them. Remind them how grateful you are for everything they are and everything they have

instilled in you. Nothing to do with Crohn's Disease, just do it.

12. Remember it's not a competition between sufferers as to who has the worst end of the diseased stick. 'Competitive suffering' is pointless and redundant. Focus on getting yourself as well as you can be and don't waste your, or others', time in bullying them into pitying you.

11. Do not tolerate or welcome pity.

10. Try not to play the victim. You have an incurable illness but that doesn't give you carte blanche to act like a complete arse when things aren't going your way.

9. Carry yourself with grace in those moments Crohn's defeats you.

8. (When you can't be graceful, do whatever you need to do behind the hospital ward curtain.)

7. Do not consider your body to be imperfect; it is a walking, talking map of everything you've done and everything you've come through over your years on the planet. Don't pick at what you consider to be flaws or beat it into oblivion with endless negativity. It's honestly no fun.

6. Have fun.

5. Listen to your body. The longer you suffer from chronic illness the easier it will become to establish

what symptoms are worth worrying about and what's *JUST A COLD*. Your body is amazing and has the capacity to tell you what it needs when it needs it. Start to pay attention to what's happening in your own skin and the answers will speak for themselves.

4. Don't waste your valuable time worrying about what other people think of you. What *you* think of you is what really matters; are you happy with the person you've become? If not, what can you do to change that? Do it.

3. Try to be tolerant of yourself and of others. Don't allow your frustration at your failing body to spill out. It will eventually destroy even the most solid of your relationships. If you're struggling, talk.

2. Love deeply and show the people who care what they mean to you whenever you can. You can't ever tell someone how wonderful they are too regularly. Although that restraining order I got in 2003 may suggest otherwise.

1. Wet wipes are, and always will be, your one true friend.

You are WELCOME.

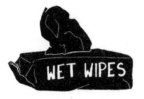

THE LOVELY CROHN'S

It's very important to try to maintain some semblance of normality in living with an abnormal illness.

For example, I always take mascara with me when I'm staying in hospital. Why? It makes me feel less unattractive and allows me to uphold some semblance of a routine. It helps make me feel I am still keeping a grip on the things I would normally do outside the confines of hospital walls.

When I've been vomiting all night and am in agonising pain, I already feel hideous and well and truly 'off' on the inside; I don't necessarily want the packaging to spoil too.

I am, of course, well aware that it's highly unlikely anyone will come to visit me and, rather than focus on all the tubes sticking out of my various orifices, comment: 'What have you done with your eyes? They look great?!' But that's not the point. It's for ME. It makes ME feel a little better about myself. It stops me from falling into a downward spiral where I don't give a hoot about myself.

You will find that most patients have something similar, something that reminds them of their life 'B.H.' (Before Hospital) and helps them keep a foot, or a beautifully curled eyelash, in the real world.

Let's face it, Crohn's is NOT a 'sexy' illness, by any stretch of the imagination. Although I must confess, I'm now struggling to think of one that is. But you get my point. Where Crohn's is concerned we have to contend with our bodies being doubled up like The Hunchback of Notre Dame when in pain, feeling and appearing bloated and suffering skin and scalp issues, nasty mouth ulcers and sore gums. Constantly running the risk of rushing to the toilet and reappearing again who knows when, etc. ETC.

These are not exactly qualities or habits traditionally associated with attractiveness or sex appeal.

I propose that this attitude needs to change; people should focus more on the incredible strength and resilience that goes hand in hand with having Crohn's. Now these qualities ARE attractive.

Although, with all that in mind, when patients are at their worst, looking good is generally further from their thoughts than the idea of never having to go to the toilet again.

The longer you spend in hospital, the longer you can start to feel detached from the world outside your own little ward. You can quite quickly find yourself feeling very isolated and it can become increasingly hard to even so much as *think* about returning to a 'normal' environment. This in itself can also be incredibly frightening. The thought of having to face things without the aid of an on-standby medical team can be a huge cause for distress. What if I take a turn for the worse? I can't just press a buzzer above my head at any hour of the day for a nurse to appear. Whether your stay in hospital is for a few days or a few months, it always tends to feel as if it's a whole new world on getting 'out'.

As the illness itself is so unpredictable, it's essential to be prepared if the need to be admitted to hospital occurs without prior warning. If I'm told to 'ward this way', I want to be ready.

A bit of pre-hospital preparation is incredibly useful in living with a chronic illness. If I'm capable, I want to ensure I make things as easy as possible for my partner, or whoever is around, to be able to get what I need brought to me as quickly as they are able. What I mean by this is that I have a 'Hospital Checklist': a list of my personal 'essential' items for a stay in hospital. It really is incredibly handy, and not in any way anal or control-freaky.

Before my Crohn's surgery, I was in and out of hospital so regularly that over time I developed a routine of keeping a pre-packed case on standby. It was a necessity, as I was causing myself unnecessary stress and panic every time I was admitted. This situation was already nerve-wracking enough in itself.

What's that? Ah yes, well since you ask, one of my top tips for hospital packing would be to pack quickly and precisely; you don't need enough for a three-week stay in the Caribbean. Although wouldn't a pina colada by a clear blue ocean be a wonderful alternative to spotted dick and curdled custard in a bleach-scented ward? Remember, you will most likely only have a tiny cupboard in which to stash your hospital bounty.

Think 'dirty weekend', with the 'dirt' being replaced by 'hand sanitizer' and the 'weekend' being replaced with 'an additional three days due to staff shortages'.

If you, like me, are partial to a hospital stay, and have been stamping that hospital loyalty card with overnight visits (one more stamp and I get to take home a hot nurse!), you should heed my top tips for hospital packing. Men: you may want to modify some of these items to suit your own particular needs.

1. **Books**. Hospitals can be boring places, so reading material can while away many a sickly hour. See also, magazines, puzzle books, jazz mags (only if you appreciate jazz, obviously).

2. **Pants**. You can never have too many clean pairs of drawers with you. Clean undies are incredibly important, particularly where bottom-related conditions are concerned. Rear-End-Freshness is next to Godliness. At least I think that's the phrase; it's a while since I read my Bible. Sanitary products too – even if it's not approaching your 'time of the month' it's always a good idea to be prepared for any potential undercarriage leakages.

3. **Pyjamas**. I typically pack two pairs initially – I usually have a fever in hospital, so heavy, thick-fabric PJs are far from pleasant. The temperature in wards can fluctuate wildly from one hour to the next, so it's hard to find a clothing balance to suit. I tend to favour long bottoms for warmth and tank tops for freshness and comfort. These styles of top are also handy for ease of application of cannulas, needles, etc. Nothing too low cut obviously, unless you are trying to seduce a doctor, which I personally wouldn't advise. It's always ended up in immediate ejection or restraining orders for me. But each to his/her own.

4. **Hairbrush**. To perform the brushing of thine hair.

5. **Deodorant**. To deodorise thine pits.

6.   **Pills**. Always remember to pack all your medication. The hospital may take these from you on admission and re-administer/refresh your prescription as you leave. It's important your doctor has a full picture of what drugs you were taking prior to admission, so he/she can best decide how to proceed.

7.   **Slippers**. Hospitals generally have cold floors and I have cold feet.

8.   **Charger/phone**. As it is almost surgically attached to me at the best of times, I think I would go slowly insane if my phone ceased to be. I would feel as if I'd lost my contact with the outside world. It's a wonderful lifeline. Also I suspect my mum would worry herself into a mild frenzy if she couldn't keep in regular contact with me.

9.   **Headphones**. Thank you for the music! I *love* music and in hospital it's certainly a million times more relaxing to listen to soothing whale music/heavy metal/Phantom of the Opera outtakes or whatever you're into than half a dozen pensioners relaying their medical woes back and forth in a game of I'm-Worse-Off-Than-You Tennis. If you have difficulty in sleeping due to the sounds of buzzers going off and various bodily cavities being excavated around you, then sometimes listening to something soothing can help aid a more restful slumber.

10. **Make-up**. Ok not *really* an 'essential', but a little blush and mascara can help to make you feel a

little more human, and it's a nice way to try to build a routine as you would at home.

11. **Lip balm**. I would not survive a day without at least two lip balms on my person at all times. No joke. My obsession aside though, it can be great to keep your lips from getting painful and chapped.

12. **Toothpaste/toothbrush**. For the freshening of that continually sickly mouth. See also: removal of the taste of unsavoury hospital food.

13. **Cat/kitten/both**. I WISH.

Another few important items worth mentioning that didn't make the list, would include a dressing gown, cash (not a lot), diluting juice (I HATE water) and a bountiful array of socks. Personal choices, I appreciate, but home comforts are very important when being away from home is forced upon you.

So there you have it, you are now so well prepared you'll be *choosing* to check in at your local hospital ASAP just to try out my list! Or maybe not. But seriously, no thanks necessary, a hamper of kittens in little bow ties will suffice.

TWO BIRDS, ONE CROHN

One of the more testing aspects of living with Crohn's Disease is opening up to your doctor and discussing your more 'intimate' areas. More importantly, what exactly goes on *down 'there'*. Although Crohn's isn't all about the rear end, the most common symptoms tend to occur in that part of the body. Therefore, and as I've mentioned previously, it's an area that has to be made, shall we say, *accessible,* in order to establish the root causes of our problems, or to appreciate the full extent of certain issues.

However, some patients find they never quite get over this apparent phobia or just general shame in talking openly about their backsides and nether regions. This is something that I've also struggled to adapt to. I have to say, I still find it difficult even now to be honest, but it's getting easier.

In most cases, the fear and anxiety in talking to doctors about your rear end (and beyond) becomes decidedly less terrifying over time. Some patients find it helpful to write their symptoms and issues down before attending their appointment. This way, they don't feel quite so bogged down in the embarrassment of the situation and can think more clearly about their questions and answers without turning 50 shades of red.

Difficulty in talking about your condition with doctors and nurses can be a major stumbling block for many when it comes to learning to adapt to your illness.

For me, I've always found it awkward explaining how I really feel. I have this oft-overwhelming paranoia I'm being seen as a hypochondriac or am massively overreacting. I do understand now that this stumbling block was probably also a factor in the length of time it took for me to be diagnosed. I suppose this is why I consistently preach to my friends and family that honesty is always the best policy when visiting the doctor. I relay this statement again and again, as I want them to learn from my mistakes and medical stumbles. I predict that eventually I will have irritated them with this mantra so much that they will no longer be my friends, so I really have very little time to get my point across.

After having had several medical professionals (and that strange man in the hospital canteen who said he knew what he was doing) investigate my every orifice, you might think that I would lose my sense of embarrassment where this topic is concerned. But for me, it's still pretty uncomfortable. Not anywhere near as much as it once was, certainly – I do now find it easier to discuss those highly attractive topics, such as the consistency of my stool and what's been happening in my back passage (what did I say about a sexy disease, eh?).

I think it's incredibly important for us, and for future generations, to be educated in much more depth in talking about bodily functions. The human body and what goes into and comes out of it shouldn't be something to be ashamed of. We shouldn't be left so ashen in discussing something that's basically an element of how we are designed.

We eat to live; we expel the digested food and water to make room for the rest. It's one of the few things we all have in common. Well, obviously, some of us find those basic body functioning requirements easier than others.

I was brought up Catholic and therefore attended a Catholic school. Here we were taught our A, B, Cs and 1, 2, 3s, but mainly the ways of Our Lord. Unfortunately, this apparently meant that when it came to learning about sex and our blossoming bodies, our education was carried out under a cloak of shame by a mortified teacher. As young women we were to be ashamed of our 'time of the month' and had to keep it secret from boys at all costs. The idea of this made me laugh even then. As if the boys in the class would somehow be so completely overwhelmed with pre-pubescent desire at the thought of us bleeding for five days a month that they wouldn't be able to control themselves. All hell would break loose. Literally. And we, as innocent and naïve young women, wouldn't have an ounce of say in the matter.

We were led to believe sex was a bad and highly uncomfortable activity – a simple tool for baby-making and nothing else. Albeit, within the boundaries of wedlock, naturally. The physical act of intercourse itself was portrayed as incredibly uncomfortable; your delicate lady area was to be pummelled and then brutally deserted without as much as a box of Milk Tray for your trouble.

Now, I don't in any way mean to belittle my education or Catholicism itself. This was just my experience and that of many people of my age. We were, unfortunately, encouraged *not* to open up about our bodies, which for me made it all the more difficult in later life. My mum was always on hand to talk to, but, again, by the time I was developing as a woman I was so filled with embarrassment about what was happening to my own body that I didn't want, or consider it helpful, to talk to anyone about it. I didn't feel the questions I had were relevant, because it would all fall into place sooner or later regardless. That was my daft teenage theory anyway.

I'd like to think this attitude has shifted, or at least dissipated, over the last 20 years or so since I was at school (*THROWS UP AT THE THOUGHT OF MY ADVANCING YEARS*) but really I'm not so sure.

Upbringing and attitudes towards your body have, I think, an immense part to play in how open patients can be, at any age. Of course, discussing such lovely aspects of Crohn's Disease as rectal bleeding, severe diarrhoea or epic gas are never going to be particularly enjoyable, for either party in the conversation, but I do believe they can become less excruciating over time.

Sometimes the simple task of 'precursoring' your conversation with the doctor by explaining how difficult you will find talking about it can help; they may, for example, try to question you in a different way or avoid certain phrases you find uncomfortable.

I find humour helps in these situations too, as unlikely as it may seem. I make stupid jokes about the ridiculousness of my situation with the doctors, mainly to shield my own embarrassment and to help me relax. This usually, in turn, evades any awkward atmosphere and makes the whole sorry situation more relaxed for everyone concerned. Although, do bear in mind this jokey method doesn't apply to all health professionals: 'You've got two months to live, LOL!' wasn't funny the last 15 times and it's still not funny now.

But in all seriousness, doctors are humans too and can pick up on an awkward situation just like the rest of us. Sometimes they can even create it!

Try to remember that although you may feel you've lost a little piece of it, you can always collect your dignity at the door on the way out again; it's not gone forever.

DISEASEY LIKE SUNDAY MORNING

I could quite honestly say that I've felt pain and discomfort in one form or another for as long as I can remember. It may seem silly to read that sentence aloud, thinking 'how could you not know there was something wrong?', but you also have to bear in mind that I had never known anything else.

I suppose, looking back, I used to think there was maybe something slightly out of the ordinary with my guts in my mid-teens, as my toilet habits seemed slightly askew. I'd alternate from regularly having diarrhoea to being constipated and bloated for weeks on end. I found my stomach could grumble on cue so substantially and so loudly that it got to the point where it had become a running party trick.

I wouldn't have dreamed of approaching a doctor with this though, as, again, how was I to know I was 'ill'? Didn't everyone's tums and bums perform in the same way?

As I left my teens and entered my twenties, my main gripe with my stomach was the way in which I was ALWAYS, without fail, full to bursting after EVERY meal. Literally jam-packed – bloated beyond compare. It didn't seem to matter how big or small the plate of food was either. I was always forced to eat tiny portions.

In fact, as a Spanish colleague once told me, 'You eat like a BIRD Kathleen! A BIIIIIRRRRRRDDDD!' (She may or may not have had anger issues...)

I couldn't understand how everyone around me seemed to be able to finish what I considered to be huge plates of food without any issues whatsoever. Some of them could even consider, and follow through with, HAVING DESSERT. Jesus. It just didn't bear thinking about.

My lack of appetite and minuscule portions of food didn't go unnoticed amongst those around me either. Some of my friends even thought I might have had some mild form of eating disorder. I can't really blame them, if I'm being honest. I'd eat no more than a few mouthfuls, complain about being full and then have to rush to the toilet. Little did they know the food was coming out of the opposite end to the one they'd possibly expected it to be.

To me, at the time, the very thought I had an eating disorder was utterly ridiculous. I loved food and the idea that I was expelling it ahead of my body's schedule, and through choice, was completely ludicrous. But I was very slim, barely ate and rushed to the loo a lot, so again I can understand entirely where they gathered these fears from. I'd never even heard of anything like Crohn's or Colitis – barely even knew what IBS stood for, so why would they assume I had anything similar either? IBS, for those unaware, is Irritable Bowel Syndrome – a common condition affecting the 'gut' causing abdominal cramping, bloating and constipation amongst others.

Looking back now, long after my diagnosis, some of my friends felt that if they had mentioned their worries and suspicions sooner I might perhaps have been treated more swiftly. But I think that's a counterproductive way to think and pretty much impossible to guess. It's very unlikely I would have taken much more action than shrugging it off, feeling insulted or reassuring them I loved my food. I really did and still do for that matter. I really do. We just have a…volatile relationship.

It really was like everything fell into place when I found out what Crohn's entailed. It was a revelation! I couldn't eat big portions because I simply didn't have the capacity! I had to cut everything into tiny pieces to try to digest it! I felt I suddenly had all the answers to questions I'd never even known needed asking. But the problem was, now that I had this information, I didn't have the first clue what to do with it.

Now, in cases where I am called upon to explain my eating habits, I almost have an excuse. No – a *reason*.

If anyone dares to query why my chicken breast has been diced into a million easy-to-manage pieces, I explain it's because I have a condition that makes it incredibly hard to tolerate and digest food.

It still sometimes makes for awkward moments in restaurants, though. Most places tend to look at you as though you don't know your own mind if you ask for a small portion or scowl like you are the spawn of Satan when they come to collect your plate on which half a plateful still remains. Waiting staff will often ask: 'Was there a problem with your meal?' or 'Didn't you enjoy it?', and I have to smile calmly and explain: 'Yes, I did, I just can't manage huge portions because I have a condition…'

But by that point they've already walked away and started serving Table 39 with the five overweight kids and the dad who looks like a big tipper.

Now I just favour replying politely with something along the lines of: 'Yes, it was delicious, just too much for me'. Either way, there's generally still an expectation on you or an air of disbelief that you just have to learn to shrug off.

It's at moments like these when it can dawn on you just how much of a part Crohn's can play in your life. Adapting to the illness is one thing, but having to consider your gut in all social situations can be quite another. Where eating out is concerned, it can be a minefield with a bowel disease. The toilets must first be scoped out, the menu scanned for potential stomach destroyers, other diners' portion-sizes investigated and the waiter befriended. Friendly waiting staff are a massive boon to an Inflammatory Bowel Disease sufferer, allowing you to be honest about why you are perhaps going to be a little more difficult than their average customer. You certainly don't need to tell them your life story – in fact, I'm pretty sure they don't want to hear it – but explaining briefly why you don't want chillies in the chilli dip might make them a little more tolerant. Or it may, at the very least, make them think twice before allowing the chef to spit in your pesto-less pesto.

A ROLLING CROHN GATHERS NO MOSS

I've chosen to accept what I have lost through my illness and focus on what I have and what positives I've gained.

This doesn't happen overnight though; it takes lots of time and even more patience and, as a certain moonwalking pop star once said, you have to start by looking at the man in the mirror.

In my case, the fact that I lack a penis and white sequinned glove aside, this meant learning to stop wallowing in my own misfortune and think about how I could learn to help *myself* deal with things outside the confines and security of a hospital ward.

Although it's obviously impossible for people with Crohn's to 'cure' ourselves, there are certain ways in which patients can help play a part in aiding their own recovery and in maintaining good well-being. Mental as well as physical that is. It's almost a requirement we have as patients to sustain as positive a level of health as we can.

For a start, it's very important you don't rely too heavily on your doctor. Remember, it's vital you are as well as can be, as often as can be, but don't assume every little issue is linked to your condition. Sometimes a cold is just a plain old cold, so treat it as such; don't dramatise things unnecessarily or jump to conclusions.

Try your best to help your doctor where you can. It's their job to help you feel as good as you possibly can. Hindering that because things are not moving as quickly as you'd like really doesn't help either of you.

If you are worried about reoccurrence of Crohn's, or about a flare-up, try to ensure your hospital or GP can arrange someone who you can call in your hour/s of need. It's a very thrilling prospect to know you have an expert in your pocket, not literally of course – technology hasn't advanced that far yet (certainly not at the time of publishing, anyway), but remember never to take advantage of it.

It can often be a huge weight off your shoulders just to know there will be someone you can call when times get tough. A lot of the stress that exacerbates Crohn's can be brought on by worry of being left to your own devices or of having to explain yourself over and over, again and again to health professionals. It can be a blessed relief not to have to repeat the whole sorry tale to a relative stranger AGAIN.

When living with a chronic illness, spending lots of time in hospital, or with your doctor, tends to come with the territory. So it stands to reason that we will often end up forming relationships with medical professionals based on (preferably mutual) trust and respect.

Your doctor must treat you with dignity and patience, whilst keeping your details confidential and preparing for consultations with as much background information to hand as they are able. The patient also has accountabilities: we are expected to be honest and open about our symptoms and to follow any given advice to the best of our ability. It's a mutually beneficial relationship that can develop well over time.

After several weeks, months and maybe years with the same doctor, these patient–professional relationships can be a massive comfort. It's incredibly reassuring as the long-suffering sufferer, to feel you are being listened to and, even more importantly, being understood. An unprepared and uninterested doctor makes for an unhappy and anxious patient.

I've been very lucky with my treatment in the years following my diagnosis. I've felt my consultants and nurses have ensured I'm well aware that help is only a phone call away. If I find I'm struggling, their support is always around me, like a stethoscope round doctors' shoulders. Although, not literally, because that would be really weird and probably break some major patient–doctor rules/laws/restraining orders.

Prior to my eventual diagnosis, I was passed from pillar to post before eventually being herded down the right path towards a viable resolution. I realise now how difficult Crohn's can be to diagnose and what a plethora of tests and procedures are normally required to get the medical mystery solved. Diagnosis is really only the beginning though. It can then take an even longer length of time to find the right form of pain management for each patient. Clearly, everyone is different and every person reacts to treatments and medications in their own unique way. This can, unfortunately, require the doctors to begin proceedings with a trial-and-error method until they make a perfect match of patient to meds. Like some warped Blind Date but with medication and patient instead of two lonely singletons (where Cilla Black fits in to this analogy, I have absolutely no idea).

How the patient reacts to these treatments can also change over the course of a lifetime, as the disease can be so changeable and, as we've mentioned, *annoyingly*, incurable.

When you are lucky enough to have someone in charge of your care who takes the time to get to know you and not treat you like simply another pest to cross off his or her list, it's a truly wonderful thing. This is why it can be so worrying when changing doctors for reasons outwith your control. It's an anxious time for any patient and can feel as if we're starting from scratch again. This can be an infuriating situation, especially if you've previously dealt with someone who knows your condition inside out (this is often literal where Crohn's is concerned).

I'm learning to be more open with my consultants; I usually find I try to make excuses for my own symptoms or find the answers so they don't have to, but the bottom line is: I'm the sick one and they are the sticking plaster. If I keep that in mind I can't go far wrong.

You may be reading this as a new patient, freshly diagnosed with Crohn's and a relatively new kid on the diseased block, still a little scared and bewildered by the thought of it all.

Or you may have a loved one who has the condition and be nervous and worried about what the future holds for them and/or how it will affect your relationship with them.

Whatever the situation, it's important to remember that although Crohn's Disease is a serious, incurable and chronic illness, it's not the end.

Your life will go on. Quite how much you allow it to change really is up to you.

3

INVISIBLE ILLNESS

STICKS AND CROHN'S

Saturday 25 September 2010

'Mum said Dad asked her "Is this operation she's getting serious?" – he's terrified of all this and I hate upsetting everyone around me, worry central round here.'

Tuesday 9 November 2010

'...yet another night of diaoherrea (I'll never know how to spell that) and vomiting...'

'HELLO. MY NAME'S KATHLEEN AND I HAVE CROHN'S DISEASE'

If the above sentence sounds as though I'm reluctantly admitting to some awful affliction, it's because although that's certainly not how *I* feel, it's often how people on the outside react when being informed of my condition.

I typically find myself faced with an unpalatable mixture of confusion, fear and pity, all peppered with a blank and vaguely disgusted expression. It's a grotesque series of faces not quite knowing where to place their features. Terrified they may somehow manage to offend me with a misplaced jaunty eyebrow.

From the beginning of my Crohn's 'career' to date, I've encountered many varied, interesting, surprising and downright bizarre reactions after divulging the finer points of my illness to others.

As a rule, I try not to overload people new to the disease with too much information. At first anyway...

I tend not to bother telling people I suffer with Crohn's unless it's mentioned by the other party or the situation requires me to. Not because I'm ashamed, by any stretch of the imagination, but because I never want to be known from the get-go as the 'sick one'. I am, and always will be, much more than my disease. So it's important to me that people know that from the outset.

Crohn's is a condition I live with, and am at times floored by, but on the whole I am still a 'normal' person. In spite of my deranged insides.

I never want to be pitied or feel I am missing out on, or being held back from, anything because of my disease.

It's essential as a sufferer that you feel in control. Mainly because as patients we often feel the absolute opposite: that our body rules everything we do. Its ignorance and selfishness can spoil our plans, stop us in our tracks (often literally) or even hospitalise us at the drop of a hat. This can be increasingly irritating and difficult for friends and family to deal with, as we are often forced to cancel plans at the last minute, or even leave during the actual event.

Many Crohn's patients feel they can't, or just won't, make plans, as they don't want to let other people (or themselves) down. This can be an incredibly dangerous cycle to fall into, as it can eventually lead to isolation and cases of crippling depression. A road we certainly do not want to find ourselves waddling down. It can be hard to fight against these feelings, as they can be so unashamedly relentless, especially in instances when the illness is pummelling you for a prolonged period of time, with seemingly no relief in sight.

In having this disease we can be made to feel we are at the mercy of our bodies and often don't have the strength to keep fighting back.

If nothing else, I feel Crohn's has given me a dose of the fighting spirit in measures I didn't have before. I can get drunk on beating this disease, because well why not? A hangover is nothing compared with a flare-up…

CLOAK AND GAGGER

Crohn's is often referred to as an 'invisible illness'.

My understanding of this phrase is that due to the majority of its symptoms taking place under the cover of the patients' skin, it can be completely unapparent to outsiders that there is actually anything wrong. You can't *see* the disease so it can go unidentified and wholly unnoticed. As the sufferer *you* can choose to reveal what's going on inside. Or not, depending on whom you're dealing with and how you feel.

My family and friends, partner, work colleagues and cats, will all profess that they know when I'm unwell simply by looking at me. They say they can tell for a variety of reasons.

My pallor changes and I become pale (and being Scottish that pretty much means see-through).

I become quiet and withdrawn.

I rush back and forward to the toilet more regularly than before.

They also mention my stance: that I become hunched over and grasp my stomach involuntarily. I liken it to going into attack mode; I am in the midst of a pummelling so I'm bracing for impact.

Understandably, this can all be pretty upsetting or even distressing for those around me, but what can I do when I'm doing all of these things without even being aware of it myself? We are in that 'pain place' when it's hard to focus on much else, so training ourselves to 'act normal' is much easier said than done. And should we even have to? Is it fair we should feel we need to act a certain way just to appease the people we love?

I am very much aware of the fact that I often find myself becoming defensive and agitated when people constantly ask me if I'm 'alright'.

I *know* this is all done out of concern, and that I should probably just learn to smile politely and nod my head to put these people's minds at rest. But sometimes, a lot of the time, I just want to scream. Audibly, as well as internally. I've often even daydreamed of somehow having the ability to touch these people and, for just as little as a split second, let them feel my pain. (*Especially* my mortal enemies. Of which I have two, since you ask.)

No, this is not a pleasant suggestion, but I hope it serves to convey, even a miniscule amount, just how intense these feelings can be when you are struggling to maintain some semblance of normality with a totally abnormal condition. If others could get a mere 'sample' of what Crohn's patients go through on a daily basis, it would make our lives a whole lot easier.

How simple and straightforward it would be to deal with medical professionals!

No unpleasant tests and procedures!

No accusations of overreacting or hypochondria!

No sniff of confusion over how serious things are!

As yet, however, this ability does not exist. Well certainly not at the time of publishing anyway; very unfortunate.

(Oh and don't even think about pinching this idea, as I've already patented it...)

I've found that this sickly cloak of invisibility can be both a curse and a blessing.

Knowing that the power to conceal or reveal your illness is in your hands can be exhilarating.

The idea that the knowledge of your disease has to come from only you can be a powerful feeling. It allows you to go about your daily ablutions (which with Crohn's can be decidedly more often than most) without anyone knowing what's really happening behind the scenes.

My manager, for example, tells me that I rarely talk about Crohn's at work or even complain when I'm in the midst of a flare-up. She gets frustrated at this. It makes things hard for her; essentially, she can't help unless I give her all the information to work with.

I'm like a jigsaw with a missing piece. Funnily enough, a lot like my insides.

I find it odd she would say this, as it always feels to me that I talk about it too much; this clearly isn't the case though. I'd wager it's likely I only feel this way because Crohn's Disease is almost constantly on my mind. I'm living with the illness and feeling its effects 24 hours a day. It's hard to push something to the back of your mind when that something constantly pokes and prods you like an annoying younger sibling until it gets the attention it craves. The only difference where Crohn's is concerned is that unlike an annoying younger sibling, you can't lock it in the cupboard until it sobs its heart out and begs for forgiveness. (We all did that with our brothers and sisters right? Right?!)

I do feel I'm slowly but surely getting better at this being honest lark though. However, I find it's often cruelly counteracted by my desire to lead a 'normal' working life. At the root of it all, I presume my lack of balls in talking more openly with my managers and colleagues stems from the fact that I don't want to be seen as the 'sick one' of the group. I don't ever want to be considered weak. I want to be the 'Chandler' from Friends. Or even the 'Samantha' from Sex and the City. Although, with decidedly less passive-aggressive humour and MUCH less passive-aggressive sexual activity.

I don't want to be known for my illness. I want to be the friendly, funny, show-stoppingly beautiful one. I know the first two will take me a wee while to perfect, but I'm certainly getting there.

ACHE, RATTLE AND ROLL

Due to the aforementioned 'invisible' aspect of Crohn's, it can very often become extremely difficult to express to those around us exactly what is going on under the surface. It can often feel very frustrating when others begin to make assumptions about what we are going through.

When I'm in the grip of abdominal pain, I often underestimate how frightening it may look to the outside world. I've had friends and family look utterly aghast and shocked and even burst into tears to see me hurting. It's very easy (and dangerous) at times for me to forget just how awful the aches that go side by side with this condition can be. In a vain attempt to make my pained appearance easier to bear for the people on the outside of my colon, I often find myself saying things along the lines of: 'Don't worry, I'm used to it!' or: 'It'll pass in a minute!'. Both of which aren't necessarily fibs – the truth is, I am, and maybe it will. But then again, maybe it won't.

I'm in pain *a lot*.

But the 'bottom line' is (* PUN CLAXON *), however disheartening it may seem, I personally don't think that as a sufferer you ever really 'get used to it'. You just learn to live with it. Adapt. Over time, your perception and management of pain changes, and you find you start to learn your own wee ways to cope. You acquire your own devices of distraction and maybe even methods to ease it.

The pain experienced by many Crohn's sufferers can at times become unbearable and almost impossible to describe. Which in itself is a bit of a waking nightmare – how can doctors be expected to help us to the best of their abilities when we can't explain the level of pain we feel ourselves?

Pain is an extremely subjective thing. One man's kick to the balls is another man's severed leg. (Obviously, I use men in this analogy, as they are generally the ones who have the balls.) Every person has a different pain threshold, and in living with chronic illness, over time, patients find themselves adapting to what they can *tolerate,* and when outside help or simply drug-induced oblivion is required.

Crohn's pain is said to be similar to that of suffering with contractions. Never having pushed out a bambino myself I can neither confirm nor deny this comparison, but I do understand where it comes from. For me, when the abdominal pain is at its worst, it normally comes in waves. Sharp, agonising spikes, akin to being viciously stabbed with a hot poker every few minutes, gradually drawing closer together until eventually I find I've arrived in Pain City without so much as an atlas.

However, the pain can also feel like a form of dull ache or cramp, akin to trapped wind or period pain but never quite the same – it's a feeling all of its own, which often makes the idea of describing it utterly redundant.

I have noticed I've gradually developed certain tics over the years that I seem to revert back to when I'm feeling at my worst.

I clench my fist. Only my right one *of course,* two would make me look like I'm *mental* and I don't want to be caught walking down the street with a screwed up face and *two* clenched fists, all kinds of hijinks could kick off. I'm certainly more of a lover than a fighter.

I try to steady and slow my breathing. Maybe the contraction comparison gave me this idea, but I've found it helps to calm me down if I get into a panic, for example, if the pain hits when I'm at my work, on the bus or doing a bungee jump. I often think: 'I'm going to throw up, I'm going to collapse' – all very unhelpful thoughts, I appreciate, but they appear regularly, so it really helps to take a minute to slow the brain down. It also works as a sort of temporary distraction from focusing purely on the pain.

I suppose I probably find it difficult to describe my pain, because I often don't appreciate just how bad it is. As mentioned earlier, it's not uncommon for me to revert back to that old 'I'm used to it' chestnut. On the other hand, just because I deal with it regularly all on my lonesome, it doesn't necessarily mean I should be putting up with it.

I believe I usually resolve to settle for what I have, pain-wise. These painkillers will *probably* do the trick for now, a day off work and I *should* be fine, a lie down and I'll *more than likely* be better in about an hour.

BUT MAYBE NOT.

Maybe I need to go the hospital, or maybe I need to see what other medication I should or could be on. But as a Crohn's patient, hospital isn't necessarily a place you want to frequent, unless it's completely unavoidable. We spend more than enough time there already.

At the end of the day, only you as the patient know your own body. Only you know what you can, and more importantly can't, endure. If it gets too much, it's vital you see someone qualified to help you. Don't be afraid of hospitals; they will always suck for a while, but at least you won't have to feel you are alone in your suffering or in the last throes of existence. Pain is, well, it's a pain. Like any other pains in your life, choose not to tolerate it.

Allow yourself to feel proud of how you deal with your disease but never too proud to seek help when you really need it.

THE CROHN RANGER

Obviously (as you may have gathered in me having written a book about it), I now personally have no qualms in discussing my chronic condition with the wider world. I am more than happy to explain all that Crohn's Disease entails to anyone who is interested enough to ask and has a stomach strong enough to listen. I'm especially chuffed if I, even in a small way, can educate people on what patients have to endure in living with the condition, and I am over the moon to be able to play even as much as the tiniest part in raising awareness about the disease.

However, one aspect of this 'openness' I'm not so overjoyed about is having to dispute often-idiotic, so-called 'facts' about Crohn's Disease.

It can be incredibly aggravating and can feel as if you are constantly batting away a pesky fly that JUST WON'T DIE.

In my short Crohn's 'career' to date, there have been many, MANY, ridiculous statements made, to me and to others, about my condition. In fact, I'd go as far as to say there are potentially too many to list in just one book (do look out for yourself in the sequel). I suppose it may seem a wee bit smug and a shade patronising now that I have knowledge of the disease to shrug these comments off or dismiss them as inane. Why should I judge other people for asking questions or making assumptions I may well have made myself a few years ago?

Because I have it, that's why.

That by no means implies I don't want anyone to talk about it. I truly do. I want anyone to feel comfortable enough to ask me anything about Crohn's – it's still a lesser-known condition, so any awareness is vitally important and goes that little bit further towards finding a cure.

I just don't want people telling ME what I'm going through based on information *they've* picked up from WebMD, or daytime TV or plucked from snippets of eavesdropped conversations.

The main example I have from this category of inane comment relates to a conversation I happened to overhear a few years ago. Two of my then colleagues were discussing my illness in a busy room. One of these seasoned gossipers was advising the other that because I have Crohn's Disease, I '…literally shit all the time'. Lovely! The person on the receiving end of this delicious nugget of information was utterly aghast with horror and mild disgust. Now please bear with me while I break this particular statement down into its component parts:

Number one: 'literally' – I 'literally' shit all the time. Really?! How do I manage to eat? And sleep? And hold down a full-time job? Surely I must be surgically attached to the toilet for fear of constant accidents?!

Number two (and I'm well aware of the irony of that): 'shit *all the time*' – again, 'all the time' – how do I manage to get anything done? (Other than the aforementioned 'shitting', of course.)

Anyway, I came back at this point in the conversation and calmly sat down to a stony and embarrassed silence. I explained calmly that, no, I don't in fact need to use the toilet all the time. I have a condition that affects my bowels and intestines, and part of the illness is a difficulty in eating and digesting, and yes sometimes expelling, foods properly. This, in turn, means that I may sometimes spend longer than your average poo-poo bear in the facilities.

My response to their general nosiness and inaccuracy just created confusion between the duo of bitchy females and those seemingly obligatory looks of pity thrown in for good measure.

These pitiful looks are also a very common occurrence when talking about your disease for the first time. (And just a heads up, they don't make us feel any better.) I know I certainly don't want anyone to feel sorry for me. I just have a condition; I haven't lost every member of my family in some kind of tragedy, like a horrific haggis-hunting accident. Again.

I'm still the same person, just minus a bit of bowel.

So, in an attempt to help YOU in coping with similar situations if and when they arise and, I hope, to stop you going down the route that will see you pick up an assault charge, here are some of my own tried-and-tested (and as polite as humanly possible) responses to some of the most common (and some of the daftest) comments/questions posed about the disease.

'You have Crohn's? So you must be at the toilet all the time?'

'No. I do have incredible difficulty in digesting food, which can mean I may have to visit the facilities more than most but, no, not "all the time". A symptom of Crohn's can be severe diarrhoea where the porcelain and I become the closest of friends, but thankfully it doesn't mean my life is spent solely in the lavatory.'

This is a popular and incredibly common misconception about the disease. As soon as bowels are so much as whispered about, people automatically assume it's simply a case of IBS (see below), intense diarrhoea or constipation you are suffering from. It's an easy fix for people. They don't want to be bamboozled with the 'incurable' patter, as it's too much to grasp. They can struggle to know what their face should do: should I pity you here? Do the tilted head and petted lip manoeuvre? Often, it seems, regardless of explaining the more complex issues related to the condition several times, people still tend to focus on the 'rear' aspect. Frustrating, yet understandable in my case – it's a mighty fine rear.

'Ah Crohn's, that's like IBS?'

'NO. IT'S. NOT. IBS is a "syndrome"; Crohn's is a disease. Irritable Bowel Syndrome can cause abdominal cramping and diarrhoea. It is generally eased by taking pain relief and avoiding certain foods. It is, on the whole, unpleasant but entirely manageable. Crohn's Disease is an IBD: an Inflammatory Bowel Disease, which can cause severe abdominal pain, rectal bleeding, bloating and swelling of the stomach and intestines, joint pain, osteoporosis, arthritis, loss of appetite, fibromyalgia, severe diarrhoea and anaemia (to name but a few) and currently has no cure. Surgery is often required in attempting to control the disease. Surgery is not necessary for IBS, unless it's to surgically remove a hot water bottle from a drama queen's grasp.'

This is one of the most infuriating suggestions I've come across and the one I've unfortunately encountered most often since my diagnosis. Not to discount IBS or any other similar issue as insignificant, of course, but it is not an incurable *disease*. It is incredibly common and can, thankfully, be easily managed.

Handling diet as sensibly as possible and taking over-the-counter pain relief are used to aid and control symptoms. IBS does not come with any other associated problems or lead to any mental health issues such as depression. Crohn's, on the other hand, can lead to a myriad of added complications.

'I wish I could be as skinny!'

'I'm "skinny" or SLIM, because I regrettably can't tolerate most foods. I often have sudden and prolonged bouts of vomiting and severe diarrhoea. I'm mainly malnourished, particularly during a flare-up, so maintaining any kind of weight is a constant battle. It is often a major challenge to eat without pain in the first place.'

At my lowest weight I was almost skeletal. My face was gaunt and you could see every bone sticking out sore thumbs around my features. My once...ahem...ample chest had all but disappeared. My hair was dry and falling out in clumps and my scalp painful and flaky. My skin was chapped and sore and I felt more unattractive than I'd ever felt. I'd dropped three dress sizes and four bra sizes. It hurt *everywhere* to so much as move because I was so painfully thin. My hair hurt (what was left of it anyway).

When I see photographs of myself from back then I feel sad and often disheartened that I may be in the same position in the future. At my lightest weight I would have given anything to have the ability to gleefully stuff my face with delicious, pain-free food. I'd have given several inches of my intestines (and I eventually did) to be able to pile on the pounds, but for Crohnies that's not always that easy. So please do not assume that losing weight is a positive for those of us with a chronic illness. For me it's a sign things are getting worse. As my weight falls off, it generally means my health is following suit and that's a slippery slope that we often don't have the energy to climb back up.

'Oh I had a relative who had that!'

'Your relative may be considered in "remission", but, unfortunately for most, such a thing doesn't exist (or in any case last very long). There is currently no cure for the disease.'

People often make the assumption that when patients tend to experience minimal or non-existent symptoms for quite some time, or have periods of what's oft referred to as 'remission', they are no longer suffering from Crohn's Disease. This, I should throw in, has never happened for me personally. It is a quite wonderful thing if these people are no longer experiencing pain or suffering from any other symptoms, but it doesn't necessarily mean they are no longer a fully paid-up member of the Crohnie Club. The disease is, at present, a lifelong condition, therefore it doesn't, and irritatingly won't, just go away. No matter how much you may beg your stomach otherwise.

It really should go without saying that periods of good health should be absolutely relished and rejoiced in, but in doing so others can often jump to the conclusion you are suddenly well. I've felt, after a break from work due to ill health for example, that telling people I feel a little better often instantaneously leads them to decide for themselves that I've come back 'cured'. Or even that whatever 'bug' or 'virus' I perhaps had is now gone. It can become increasingly difficult to explain your diseased situation when those around you have already made their minds up and jumped to several wrong conclusions. But then again, why should we have to?

(★ RECOILS ★) 'Oh is it contagious?'

'No. But ignorance is.'

This particular response to disclosing the existence of your disease is probably one of the most irritating and downright insulting. That's whether it's intended that way or not. The implication there, for a start, is that you are knowingly putting others at a risk of 'catching' your disease. I suppose in many way's it's understandable that people may initially be wary when they first hear the word 'disease', but recoiling in horror or visibly cowering away from you is really not the most sensitive way to go about airing your concerns. If you must ask, then please do it in a more delicate manner. Or just do ten seconds of research.

'But you look so well?!'

'Thank you! But unfortunately I'm still sick. And next time please take the "but" out of that sentence – it'll make it sound more like a compliment than an accusation.'

This seems harmless and may even be considered a 'nice' thing to say. But to someone with Crohn's Disease, this can be unbearably maddening.

Again, it almost implies that the disease is being exaggerated in some way; it has an accusatory tone of 'how *can* you be ill?' to it. This is always a sore point for patients, as it often feels as if it is a constant battle for us to express just how bad we truly feel on the inside.

People may accuse you of 'faking it' because you look well as far as they are concerned. The illness itself being 'invisible' means you really do have to open up verbally about how you feel – in some circumstances, whether you want to or not. At times you don't even have the energy left to talk about it. The very last thing a patient really wants to do when they are in pain is to focus on it by describing their suffering in detail to others. But sometimes we, as the unfortunate minority, have to accept it can be an unpleasant necessity.

'I feel terrible too, I've got diarrhoea so I know exactly how you feel.'

'No, no you don't. You've got diarrhoea because you chose to eat that dodgy curry even after reading on the label it was a month past its sell-by date. It will pass in 24 hours. I have an incurable illness that I will most likely suffer from for life.'

Once again this is utterly *rage-inciting* patter. How can you begin to compare diarrhoea to what I have?! It's rude and shows an exasperating lack of knowledge. It makes my blood boil but can also be put down to complete ignorance on the part of person with the supposedly aching botty.

But before we start painting placards, burning our pants and taking to the streets to riot at the injustice of these comments, we should try to remember that if people are genuinely interested (and willing to listen) we could always use these opportunities to educate them a little. Crohn's isn't just about the rear end; the symptoms are vast, all encompassing and spread across the whole body in most cases. Try to express that as best you can rather than letting the rage of comments like these consume you. No need to end up serving jail time. AGAIN.

'You should just try not to let yourself get stressed…'

'Thanks for that, great suggestion! But in that same vein you should try not to make inane comments until you know what you're talking about.'

It is true that stress and anxiety are commonly known to exacerbate Crohn's symptoms, however it's not simply a case of cutting stress out of your life (if this is even at all possible). To suggest to someone with a chronic illness that they should simply 'stop stressing' is akin to advising someone with depression to just 'snap out of it'. Regardless of how much you try, life, as it is, simply does not allow for zero stress. Work pressures, relationships, money worries and just existence in general can all build up and snowball rapidly out of control. When that moment occurs, pain can strike like Bruce Willis: WITH A VENGEANCE.

There are many ways in which stress can be reduced, and techniques can be learned to help limit stressful experiences. But often with Crohn's Disease as much as a sniff of stress or anxiety can linger for hours to days, regardless. Sometimes the body just can't catch up with the brain.

'So do you have to eat a special diet?'

'Not necessarily. Many patients cater their diets to suit or in an attempt to appease their Crohn's. For some, liquid diets are required to get symptoms under control. There isn't one diet to suit all, as everyone tolerates food in their own way.'

Granted, this one is a bit of a long-winded answer and the poser of the question will probably have already left by the time you've gotten to the point, but the original response still stands.

The trick in eating with Crohn's Disease lies in finding out what foods and drinks are wrong for you. Yes, you could of course argue ALL OF THEM, but that thought process never helped anyone. There are certain foodstuffs that tend to be common 'triggers' for most patients, but over time you will find your own way in terms of what to avoid and what to devour like there's no tomorrow. Myself, I've had to cut out red meats and most dairy, as those cause me the most difficulty in terms of digestion and are well-known pain culprits. Everyone tolerates foods differently, which is why it can be so problematic to find a one-size-fits-all diet for the condition.

'You are ill again? You were sick a couple of weeks ago.'

'I'm always ill. I have an incurable illness, which means I have a condition that will flare up at any given time. So at times I may feel (and look) worse than others.'

This is another particularly frustrating statement and one that I personally tend to encounter on a regular basis. People on the outside of your intimate circle (* COUGHS *) only see you a small percentage of the time. The situation usually occurs as those on the outside – colleagues, employers, etc. – notice when you are ill. It's newsworthy. I don't even intend that to be meant badly, it's just a fact. It's annoying when people question the fact that, yet again, you are poorly.

When someone looks as awful as we typically do when a flare-up strikes, it sticks in the mind of others. Therefore, if you are ill consistently, it isn't considered 'normal'. People can't compute. Most folks have a bug, the flu or a virus and then after time it clears and they go back to living their life illness free. For Crohnies, that situation doesn't arise. We can have periods of remission or feeling 'well', but in most cases these blessed moments don't last very long.

THE BOTTOM LINE

Essentially, everyone with Crohn's Disease is different. No two patients' experiences are the same. It stands to reason that there are similarities in all cases, but each person 'suffers' differently. Much like humans themselves, each 'Crohnie' is also completely unique in their pain.

Crohn's is a very serious illness that can be Hell on Earth to live with. It's not feasible to come to your own conclusions as to what someone is going through purely by hearing their 'label' of Crohn's Disease.

It's also incredibly vital to us that you don't discount the disease as unimportant simply based on your own lack of knowledge on the subject. Please, ask! We won't bite! We also won't spontaneously excrete ourselves at the mere mention of it.

Too much time is spent pussyfooting around or jumping to conclusions where the condition is concerned. On the whole, most patients are open, willing and well prepared to discuss their situation. I think a lot of that hush-hush attitude comes from the lack of information surrounding the disease in the public domain.

It's widely considered an 'embarrassing illness'. For me, the main 'embarrassment' lies in having to explain my condition again and again to people who merely hear the word 'poo' and practically die of cringe-itis on the spot. Actually I find the phrase 'embarrassing illness' an embarrassment in itself – why in this day and age are we still 'embarrassed' about our own bodies? It's a sad state of mind that won't change until we accept that everyone is intrinsically the same. Body issues are only an embarrassment if you allow them to be viewed that way.

Many patients themselves have little to no knowledge of the disease until they are actually diagnosed. Then it's a rapid-fire questioning session with the doctor and a case of going into web search overdrive to gain more insight. As patients, on the whole we had to quiz to find out what it was, so there is probably an inbuilt urge in us now to educate others who are on the outside looking in.

Of course it stands to reason that there are some Crohnies who don't want to talk endlessly about their illness. This I can certainly understand, as I often feel this way myself. I regularly want to forget for a little while and just become 'normal'. It may sound slightly odd but when you are feeling good and symptom free, it can take something as little as a niggling stomach cramp or a bit of indigestion or trapped wind to remind you how bad things can truly be.

This in turn can be a depressing thought and perhaps eventually allow dark thoughts to creep in.

I've seen myself get dressed up for a night out, feeling attractive and confident, and then catch a glance of my swollen stomach in the mirror and think: 'What's the point?' I've already played every potential conversation over in my mind and mentally lived through every awkward question I may have to bat away, and by the point where the cogs in my head slow down I've already cancelled the taxi and pulled my heels off.

You have to try your absolute best to rise above these feelings. Hard as it may be, you cannot hide yourself away; if not only for those who care for you but for yourself. You only have one life and although it can feel difficult and utterly exhausting at times, you have to continue to live it. Diseased or not.

My partner, for example, is forever telling me to make the most of myself. He tells me he won't hear of me recounting regrets when we are old and grey. He reminds me I am beautiful in his eyes and should enjoy that fact and stop covering up; be proud of what I have. All wonderful advice, but it's often mind over matter. I KNOW what he's saying is true (well I'm TRYING to believe the 'beautiful' bit…), but when I feel low and can't see a way out it's hard to see things quite as positively as he does.

I try to stop and look through his eyes, but unfortunately he often finds the eye-swapping surgery too time consuming and painful.

I try to think how I would feel if I could see him allowing an illness to hide his light. I would be sad beyond belief, because he is the most amazing man I've ever met. I wouldn't be able to see him beat himself up without it breaking my heart.

So, I try my best to look on the bright side of life, even when my guts try to keep me in the gloom.

Like most sufferers, it's understandable that I have many spells when I absolutely HATE my illness.

My romance with my aforementioned partner aside, somewhat confusingly, I have another 'relationship' running parallel.

I have what you could call a love–hate relationship with my colon.

We have the trickiest and at times most volatile of relationships, yet we endure. I often mentally compare my gut to an awkward and needy boyfriend. The type who wants to be involved in *everything* I do. Then has major tantrums when he doesn't get his own way. SO BORING.

I have to consider my gut wherever I go and in whatever I do. This can be intensely irritating and can be a stark reminder of just how much this 'invisible' condition feels entirely visible.

My reluctant partner, the Gut, decides when we leave early from parties and tells me, in the most insolent manner, what I should and shouldn't be eating. He then makes me pay for disobeying him later in the evening. There's no romance here, as he regularly leaves me doubled up in pain and begging for pain relief. You could say it's a pretty toxic relationship I'm trapped in.

Sometimes that 'invisibility' factor can make me feel incredibly alone.

On the plus side though, I can hide my dodgy 'partner' from the outside world. I can ensure I don't let my bad gut affect the lives of those around me.

This invisibility makes for a happy hiding hole from my illness at times. I don't want to spend all day everyday thinking about my gut. Who wants to spend *every waking minute* thinking about a relationship?! NO ME THAT'S FO' SHO'!

Besides, I have enough framed colonoscopy pictures on my desk at work to keep those memories alive.

HERE I GO AGAIN, ON MY CROHN

Another strange aspect in living with this 'invisible' disease is what I describe as 'Competitive Suffering'. This is a very odd scenario indeed. This commonly occurs in either people who have the disease or perfectly healthy people who feel some bizarre form of jealousy. They tend to express these peculiar tendencies by assuming the symptoms of a patient in order to get sympathy or attention. I've unfortunately come across both of these in my short Crohnie career and, I have to say, I still don't really understand it. Why someone would *want* to be pitied beggars belief. I want to be known for my personality, for who I am as a young(ish) woman and how I appear to others – NOT as a patient and patient alone. It's borderline insanity and living your life as though you are a 'sick person' can only end in misery. Most likely due to the fact that I myself suffer from the condition and know all too well what it entails, I can't begin to imagine what these HEALTHY people are thinking.

Crohn's is, in essence, a horrendous illness to live with.

I hold down a full-time job with this chronic illness. I certainly don't mention this because I expect any thanks or praise for it – if I'm able to work of course I will; I need to learn a living and would never take advantage of our welfare system knowing I'm able – I just mean to express that although I am working, it doesn't mean it's not a struggle for me on a daily basis to even so much as get out of bed in the morning. I'd love to have the luxury of not having to suffer from anxiety about work and tiring myself out and worrying about bills. I'd also love to not have had a piece of my body cut out in order to save my life, but that's life. *My* life.

I understand, as I've come across it at various times in my life, that some people find it a way of life to tell tall tales and/or elaborate on illnesses they do not have. If they have felt unwell at any point, the facts of their period of incapacity will be embellished to within an inch of their lives. These people think that being in poor health will somehow give them some sort of leg up in life; perhaps get them the attention they so desperately crave. Or, and this is the one I'll never personally understand, gain the pity of those around them. Maybe I'm just getting cynical, but never at any point in my life has any good experience ever come from being pitied.

Now, for those of you who may be familiar with this strange behaviour but perhaps unfamiliar with the reality of being sick 24/7, let me tell you a little bit about what it's like to live in pain on a daily basis. Here is a short (and far from sweet) insight into the first few hours of the day for a patient with an incurable illness.

> **6.00 am:** Wake up and rush to the toilet. This will be about the fifth time I've been already this morning. I often worry I've had an accident in the night, although thankfully this has never happened to me (yet).

> **6.20 am:** I brush my teeth and shower. This hurts. Everything hurts. It hurts because my gums ache constantly from the ulcers and swelling I get when I have a flare-up. My bones ache because of the Crohn's-related arthritis I have and the joint pain I suffer constantly. It hurts to wash my hair because it

falls out in clumps and this stings my scalp. My skin prickles all over because it gets dry and painful when I feel at my worst.

6.40 am: I take a few minutes to calm down and regain my strength because I'm now hot, dizzy and faint from having been upright for so long. I'm shattered because it seems there isn't enough sleep in the world to satisfy me, so I'm fairly weak at the start of most days.

6.45 am: I get dressed and paint my face. Usually thinking all the while that this is a fruitless exercise because I'm so pale and feel utterly lifeless and that how I feel inside is written all over my face. Also my skin is usually atrocious when I'm at my worst – dry and chapped – so it can sting my eyes to adorn them with any make-up.

7.00 am: I think about breakfast. I make myself a cup of tea then rarely drink more than two sips of it because I know I'll have to rush to the toilet again and I certainly can't risk needing to 'go' when I'm on the bus to work. I think about whether or not I can tolerate food and what the consequences would be if I had a piece of toast. Will I need to throw up in ten minutes' time? Will I have to go to the toilet in twenty minutes? Can I safely time both of these activities before I leave? By the time I've been through all these possible scenarios in my head I've almost missed the bus.

Basically, my morning is mostly based around my colon and meeting its every diseased whim.

I won't bore you all by yapping on about the remaining 20 odd hours in my day. But that was just a wee snippet of what my day is like before I even leave the house in the morning.

I feel tired all the time. I feel sore and achy all the time. And I feel pain of some description ALL. THE. TIME.

If you know, or are, someone who is lucky enough to get through the day without feeling like a limp rag on a daily basis, please don't allow yourself to pretend you are hard done by. You have a life, so kindly live it. Don't waste it by wishing yourself in my or any other poorly person's shoes, because, believe me, they won't suit you. I have impeccable taste (and tiny feet).

Spending your life wallowing in misery is both incredibly unhealthy and unbelievably unappealing.

Maybe it's because I know just how precious good health can be that I feel so strongly about this, but it's heartbreaking to see people around me openly squander something I try so hard to achieve on a daily basis: *normality*.

Allow yourself to enjoy your existence and don't unwittingly insult others by implying you know what they are going through. Just listen and, if possible, 'be there'. Don't absorb problems as though they are your own.

People don't tolerate lies for long. It's important to remember how hard it ACTUALLY is for people dealing with genuine difficulties like a chronic illness. Please don't pretend you have the first clue what they are going through if you don't.

Myself, I might look sickly and frail at times, I may rely on medication and pain relief to get me through the day, but I have fighting spirit in doses I've never been prescribed before.

IBD AND SYMPATHY

When you begin, slowly, to come to terms with your new situation, you may, as I did, tentatively begin to dip your toes into the world of social networking.

With little more than a quick web search, you will find that there is a massive world of support for fledgling Crohnies out there. What can be slightly more difficult is pinpointing the right avenue of support for you as an individual.

I'd say I've personally been an active member of the online Crohn's 'community' (Twitter, Facebook, blogging, etc.) for several years now. I first started looking into avenues of support outwith my immediate and more tangible circle shortly after my surgery. I was home alone recovering most of each day and bored out of my wits. Both my brother and partner suggested I think about starting a blog. I did, quite hesitantly, but before I kicked off my own writing I did a fair bit of research. A few of the same names cropped up again and again and I felt this new arena to be a little intimidating and perhaps even a little cliquey. I didn't want to feel as if I was the new kid in the diseased playground so I initially kept my distance. But soon I found Crohn's sufferers had somehow come across my blog themselves and were following *me* and even offering the diseased hand of friendship. This in itself was incredibly encouraging. Having the reassurance from people outside of my immediate family that I was not rambling a lot of nonsense was hugely encouraging. I decided to keep on trucking with the blog and to my amazement my readership grew and grew. I've since made a few solid and wonderful bonds with fellow Crohn's sufferers from all across the globe that I can confidently say I treasure as much as my 'real-life' friendships.

When I was first diagnosed with Crohn's I entirely scoffed at the very idea of so much as speaking to anyone with the same illness as myself. The mere thought of it seemed abhorrent to me. I'm not entirely sure why this was; I think I was mainly in denial that anything was wrong with me in the first place, let alone prepared to hear more about it from someone who has had it for a lifetime. It's a pretty strange feeling to explain to someone who has never experienced such a diagnosis. It was easier for me to attempt to focus purely on getting out of hospital and not really think much further beyond that. It was too hard to deal with the idea I wasn't ever getting better. At least that's how I felt at the time. Reverse rose-tinted spectacles if you like.

Social networking is an amazing outlet for people living with chronic illness and specifically those affected by conditions that can make it completely impractical, or impossible, for them to leave their home. It can be a lifeline to the outside world and a wonderful way to develop friendships and build a support network. For those reasons and many more, I would never bad-mouth these methods of support.

However, I do feel they can, in some cases, be used negatively, which only ends up doing more harm than good. Those who use these forums as a support network or community (and I would certainly consider myself amongst them) can have often vastly different expectations. Many assume that simply having the same condition instantly establishes a bond. In my not-so-humble opinion, this is not always the case. Please do not misconstrue what I mean by this; I am more than happy to help anyone who may be suffering in any small way I can: offer advice, a listening ear, a virtual shoulder to cry on or even a giggle if at all possible. But Crohn's Disease and all its difficulties and foibles are only a PART of my life. Crohn's is not, and never will be, *all I am.* If that means that I am somehow in the wrong for not devoting more of my time to the disease and to the devotion of a Crohn's 'community' then so be it – everyone is entitled to their opinion and mine's just as valid as the next diseased person's. I like to think it's advisable to dip in and out of a community of this sort without being reprimanded or frowned upon for such an activity. I really don't think it's particularly 'healthy' for people struggling with their own well-being to spend all day every day talking, tweeting and posting about their woes. I know this because I've done it. Many times! However I imagine it would be horrifically mind-numbing if I were to post every tweet and every update about my life with Crohn's Disease. I personally can't think of anything worse. I've been lonely in hospital and bored in bed with a sick bowl, but on the few occasions I've told the world and its wife about it, I've just felt a wee bit daft and a big bit pitiful. So when I find myself feeling that way I tend to stay away from my phone or write a blog. And often not go on to publish it until I've read it back post-drug-fuelled pain haze. By which time it usually repulses me so much it ends up in that big electronic wastebasket in the sky.

Some sufferers who partake in social networking also fall into the aforementioned 'competitive suffering' category. They will want to reprimand you or remind you that they are worse off than you. This absolutely infuriates me and I feel it's incredibly harmful, especially for newly diagnosed Crohn's patients. When I first researched my own 'new' condition, I found any aspect of it online to be almost solely negative: forums professing you will surely die and how AWFUL your future will be if you do manage to grasp some semblance of a life with your bony hands. Not really what I was looking for. The hearts, flowers and unlimited loo roll aspect wasn't there in the slightest. It made me fearful to open up and talk about myself. Mainly because…are you INSANE? THAT'S TERRIFYING?! and because there can be such unparalleled jealousy and competitiveness in the medical world.

If you've ever had a stint in hospital you will know that there's always, ALWAYS one patient who is 'sicker' than you. Wasting your time trying to advise that person you are on death's door will fall on (probably profoundly) deaf ears. It can be irritating and infuriating and put you off your reheated ham sandwich.

It's completely unnecessary. Who in their right mind feels the need to compete with another sick person? That sentence itself confirms how utterly ludicrous it is.

If people are suffering then let them suffer without fear they are going to be patronised or told how to behave. Your pain is not the same as Mrs Smith in Bed 5. So don't tell her how to feel. And please don't tell her she shouldn't be complaining just because you aren't. Just carry on feeling comfortable in your own pain-beating achievements like the brave little soldier you are.

Of course, this is by no means a one-size-fits-all scenario; on the other side of the coin there are those who love to wallow in the abject misery of their lives and constantly gripe about the diseased hand the big guy has dealt them. Those people are unhappy and CHOOSE to be unhappy. I can't get with that. Leave them to it if you can't help and don't let them pull you into it.

I've found it difficult at times to deal with these individuals, as I can forget that, illness or not, people are still people. They don't suddenly become angelic and almost godlike because they are suffering. It's not the 1900s and we are NOT angels.

What I mean by this is that, Crohn's or no Crohn's, people can still be callous, rude and presumptuous. It took me an almost embarrassingly long time to realise that those people are not people I want to know at all *in life,* so why should I make space or allowances for that behaviour just because we share an illness in common? It is utterly nonsensical.

I like to think that people are still, essentially, good. I was brought up to believe that the Big Good Guy (with the white beard who sits on clouds) always beats the Big Bad Guy (with the red skin, goatee and tail) so I think in the grand scheme of things we'll all be ok in the end. (Just to avoid confusion, I'm obviously talking about Jim and Bill from my old neighbourhood there, by the way.)

On the whole, I think nowadays the good vastly outweighs the bad in the world of Crohn's support. The disease is becoming much more well known and as we progress in learning more about it there is wider scope for educating others. The best advice I can give is to take your time in researching what support is right for *you* personally. Don't just jump headlong onto the first available bandwagon. Open up and allow people to see a little of you and you'll probably find you'll be surprised at the results. There are wonderful people in the world with massive, generous hearts; just don't expect too much too soon from the kindness of strangers.

Don't ever doubt that, personally, I absolutely want to know, strangers or not, that you are all well so I can rejoice and be happy for you. I want to know you are struggling so I can try my very best to help in any way I can, but I really don't (and I'm sure I'm not alone in this) want to know the graphic details of your every bowel movement. I have more than enough of my own to contend with thank you very much.

4

RELATIONSHIPS

ROMANCING THE CROHN

Saturday 13 November 2010
'This liquid diet is KILLING me. Everyone at work chowing down on burgers today while I downed a Bovril like some poverty-stricken football fan. So RAGING.'

Sunday 30 January 2011
'Mum and Dad visited today, an hour really flies when you haven't seen a familiar face all day. I'm getting better and not blubbing when they leave now! James in at night and he said he'd slip pillows in the bed and sneak me out if I wanted. I WISH.'

THE THRILL IS CROHN

I often try to remember that although I'm the patient, I'm certainly not the only person that this disease can affect.

It can often be much harder than it may initially seem to detach yourself from your own condition and take a good look at how it must affect those around you.

Regardless of whether you would like it to be, Crohn's is *always* there. The disease can be an immense irritation for someone who tries their best to live life to the full. A patient's work life, social life and even romantic life can all take a dip from time to time due to the intensity, relentlessness and general unpleasantness of their symptoms. Unfortunately, during these 'dips' you may find you are all but helpless to avoid it.

The condition always generously makes itself known within relationships too. Crohn's is the big fat diseased gooseberry when you are out on a date with your partner. It waddles around embarrassingly and awkwardly when you are out dancing with friends. It trails behind like a geriatric pensioner when you are out doing a spot of shopping. Oh, and Crohn's just loves to lie about on the sofa like a bloated pig while housework needs attending to. You get the general idea.

This all means that the condition needs to be considered by both patient AND their loved ones in almost everything they do. Infuriating and incredibly annoying. Previously simple tasks or short trips can now require mammoth planning and almost military precision.

These comparisons got me to thinking about the other, rather intimate, love affair I have running concurrently with the one I have with my beloved…that being my aforementioned, and volatile, relationship with my Gut. It's a torrid romance we have. With so many ups and downs, we are considered by many (no one) as the Burton and Taylor of our day.

The bottom line (pun ALWAYS intended) is that my life would be a considerable extent easier if I didn't have Crohn's Disease. I would be free from worry (well, health worries anyway) and the pain and misery it can bring. I'd be able to do my own thing without having to consider how my guts will react first.

But then the same could be said of any relationship.

When things are difficult, that's all you can focus on. In the midst of anger and upset you can forget the positives in the blink of an eye. The difference between most human relationships and the one I happen to have with my gut is that we didn't have a choice in our being flung together. It was preordained. Destiny. Written in the genes, if you will. Like some awful arranged marriage where a mere two weeks in you realise that you are just NOT compatible.

Regardless, I love the bones of my gut. (Yes, I know that doesn't work but let's just go with it…)

If my disease and I were ever to be parted, I think in a way I'd miss what Crohn's has given me.

Everyone, including myself, wants a cure for the illness, and if that day ever arrives within my lifetime I'm pretty sure I will grab it with both hands. But, strangely, I also think I'd feel a great sense of loss at what we've been through together.

I don't like to consider my condition as in any way poisonous or massively negative. Not anymore, anyway. However, that doesn't mean it's easy to live with. Far from it, in fact; it's painful, stressful, and daunting and can be lethal. But like any long-term relationship, I like to think it has good points along with the bad.

If Crohn's were ever to 'leave' me, I'd want to look back on what I've gained and not spend my new-found bowel freedom focusing on what I'd lost or missed out on during our time together. Much like the conclusion of a romance with any former flame, after the dust had settled I'd try to take the time to see what good (if any) we've done one another. It's never particularly healthy to hold on to anger and bitterness at the end of any relationship, however difficult that may be to shake off.

Plus, I know for a FACT that my Crohn's Disease would never take my David Bowie CDs and 'forget' to return them.

SWORD IN THE CROHN

Although my loved ones never air any gripes they may have (and I don't doubt for a second they must have them), when it comes to 'caring' for me, I imagine it must be incredibly gruelling at times having to be the friend/mother/lover of a Crohn's patient.

Caring for someone with a chronic illness such as Crohn's Disease can be intense, sporadic and extremely unpredictable. It requires vast amounts of kindness and often boundless patience. Not because we are difficult patients you understand, but because often Crohn's is a decidedly unwelcome houseguest. One who turns up to the party uninvited and causes so much awkwardness that we have to leave early. Thankfully for me, I've discovered that the vast majority of my friends and family and my partner have this particular patience in abundance.

'Being there' for someone with this disease is not necessarily all about mopping up sick, cleaning the toilet and dabbing a fevered brow (although these activities may be required from time to time; please ensure you check the small print). It's more about learning to adapt, and helping the patient adapt, to their new situation.

It also requires you to be brutally honest from time to time. This is mainly because feeling consistently below par can cause someone with Crohn's to feel dejected a LOT of the time, so it's important to surround yourself with people who have a par big enough to tell you exactly when to snap out of it and quit wallowing. After allowing you the apt amount of wallowing time, obviously.

It's equally important, as the patient, to accept and appreciate that those individuals who love you would never intentionally set out to upset or embarrass you, so try to accept, or at least listen, to their advice with good grace and treat it with the respect it deserves.

Yes, *even* if that advice feels to you like nothing but tawdry nonsense.

On breaking the news to my friends and family that I had finally been diagnosed with Crohn's Disease, their initial and chief reactions were those of sadness, shock and confusion. Very much like myself, few of them knew anything, or they knew very little, of the condition prior to my diagnosis, therefore they had no idea what I would be dealing with. What their daughter, partner, sister and friend would be facing in the next few months and in the years to come.

When my treatment was well underway, and on discussing my condition at a later date, it transpired that a good few of my close family and friends had initially thought that Crohn's Disease was considered terminal. That I would die. How awful. I can't begin to imagine what a frightening thought that must've been, to suddenly assume you are losing your loved one. You see, without tooting my own horn too much, I am one hell of a catch and all round good gal (* INSERT SALACIOUS WINK HERE *).

In all seriousness though, this is something that still upsets me to this day: what the people I love went through, and are still going through, in living with and loving someone with a chronic illness.

Without intending to sound too dramatic, I think it's fair to say that pretty much everyone I'm close to has had their lives turned upside down to a certain extent following my own diagnosis.

The main individual being the man I share a life with and who also happens to have my heart.

Allow me to wax lyrical about him for just a moment…

The man I love is strong and proud. He is unfathomably handsome and witty, makes me laugh until I am begging for mercy and has an innate ability to perk me up when I am feeling down. Which, as most Crohn's patients know, may often be more than most.

I love him endlessly for everything he is and everything I know he will become. I feel him around me like a beautiful safety net when life makes me feel as if I am falling. He is brave and bold, sensitive and gentle and there for me whenever I need him. He, through some wonderful hiatus of rational thought, fell for me too. This happened pre-disease and, wonderfully, he still cares for me now, Crohn's and all. I believe love is enduring and, much like Crohn's itself, relentless. It doesn't quit if you are having a bad day, are shattered or spending two solid hours on the loo, AGAIN.

When I was initially diagnosed with this disease, I was so low I just took it as read that my beloved would want to leave, that our relationship would be over, and I wouldn't for a second have blamed him for it. I felt worthless and unappealing. I felt that as my future was so bleak, why should I drag the man I love through this misery with me too? What could I possibly offer him for the remainder of our years together when I'd be otherwise occupied fighting an internal war against a condition that I seemingly had no hope of winning. For someone who had no major signs of low self-esteem prior to my diagnosis, suddenly I became full of self-loathing almost overnight.

However, instead of packing his bags and booking the next flight to Outer Mongolia, my partner hugged me and simply told me that we would find a way to get through it. Instantly restoring my faith in love, and in myself, with the use of a few simple sentences and giving me the courage to fight for my health and my future. *Our future.*

(Besides, I'd already swallowed the key to his handcuffs and destroyed his passport so he didn't really have much choice in the matter.)

The man I love believes in ME and what I will, and can, become. Diseased or otherwise. When I feel like throwing everything away in a fit of anger or sadness I feel him gently giving me a kick up the backside and telling me to stop wallowing. Albeit metaphorically. Anyone with Crohn's will know that a kick in that area is always a brave move... He's certainly 'gutsy' (* PUN CLAXON *).

As much as patients like me may like it to, love can't, of course, change that fact that we have Crohn's Disease. But it can help to soothe a worried mind, ease an aching body and make you feel that you have absolutely everything to be grateful for.

I personally feel that having Crohn's has helped me to see just how important the love of my partner, my friends and my family is to me and how very important it is to always remind them of that fact. A LOT. To the point where it becomes a bit weird, creepy and uncomfortable and I hold them all a little too long and a little too tight and receive yet ANOTHER restraining order.

When I stop to consider others and how my condition affects those I care about most, it allows me to focus on what's really important. Love and happiness – for myself and for those I love. Comfort – knowing you have people around you who care and support you can be a blessed relief and a massive weight off your diseased shoulders. Living with this illness can be so all consuming at times that even having people to talk to openly and without judgement can really help. Family and friends can be amazingly useful from the base levels of giving you a hug or a friendly ear to consoling you when you have bad news or perhaps even nursing and caring for you when you are at your lowest. These are the things only people who love you (and qualified professionals getting paid for it, obviously) can and will do. Not out of some misguided sense of responsibility, or due to feelings of pity towards you, but solely out of love.

DISEASEY RIDER

For me, one of the keys to maintaining successful relationships when living with a chronic illness is honesty. It's completely essential you ensure you are in a position where you are able to revel in the comfort of talking to someone about what you are going through. This might be anyone, from a parent or lover to a friend or colleague. It's incredibly important you have a confidante of some description, as it can be surprising, and somewhat disheartening, to discover just how much Crohn's can affect you mentally as well as physically.

Knowing you have, and will have to live with, an incurable disease can cause you to get bogged down in spending time focusing on what you will lose or will have to sacrifice, rather than relishing what you still have.

Using my own situation as an example, one of my main worries when I was first diagnosed was the unrelenting fear of losing 'me' to the disease – somehow becoming less of a woman or potentially looking as unattractive as I felt and decidedly unappealing to the man I share my bed and my body with. It may perhaps sound trite or unimportant to those without a long-term condition like Crohn's, but these are all very natural and incredibly common worries amongst Crohn's sufferers, and sufferers of any chronic illness, of all ages, sexes and marital statuses.

For those people not in relationships at the point of diagnosis and beyond, the concern is often that they won't be able to attract a prospective 'mate'. They worry they don't feel, or won't be perceived as, 'sexy'. Or that they won't be much of a 'catch' for a potential partner, with bowel issues tagging along for the ride. They can feel under pressure when they do start dating someone new to reveal their disease to their beau – when is the right time? How will they react? Will the relationship survive Crohn's acting as a third wheel.

People already in relationships can become frightened that the disease will somehow change something between them as a couple. Many fear things drifting between them, possibly both sexually and emotionally. They can, quite understandably, worry that their relationship will crumble under the additional strain of one half of the twosome being the 'ill' one for the rest of their years together.

Intimacy in relationships can be another worry, along with how to adapt to having a different collection of issues to consider where the bedroom is concerned. I'm not talking painting and decorating here (unless that's what the kids are calling it these days).

I am categorically NOT going to go into any detail about my own boudoir antics, as, even in his advancing years, there is still a chance my dad will take the time to read this. If that day comes, he does not want nor need to read about his only daughter doing anything riskier than hand holding.

There are many reasons why sex and intimacy can be 50 shades of a grey area for those living with IBD (and chronic illness in general). Along with the basic initial difficulties in feeling the 'urge' due to pain, bloating, depression, exhaustion and a plethora of other issues, there are also mountains of physical issues we often have to navigate through before even considering getting our paws on our partner. So here I'll run through a few of the most common issues and some potential fixes to let you get back to business…on your back, or otherwise.

STRESS

For anyone, sickly or not, stress is a very common problem and/or reason for avoiding or simply not wanting sex. For men, sex can often be a stress *reducer*, but this is rarely the case for women. Dealing day to day with a chronic illness on top of everything else in life – work, family, home commitments – can be utterly overwhelming, so it stands to reason that doing the horizontal cha-cha is about as far from your mind as enjoyment is to a colonoscopy. In order to feel aroused, you have to be receptive; stress can hinder this, so it's important to try and work out what your biggest stressors are and focus on how to reduce them. Then cha-cha to your heart's content.

DEPRESSION

Certainly for women, depression can make our libidos sink lower than a worm's bra strap. Unfortunately, most antidepressants can have the same effect – decreasing our serotonin transmitters, which play a massive role in arousal. You know, the same happy feelings we get when we meet a new kitten or find an unopened jar of Nutella in the cupboard. Although often vital, drugs to ease depression can also decrease libido, hinder ability to orgasm or even interfere with sexual function. If this is your Achilles heel, then first stop isn't jumping off a cliff with frustration, but seeing your doctor to discuss changing medication to something with fewer side effects and/or to counteract the worst effects for you.

NEGATIVE BODY PERCEPTION

With all IBD can do to our bodies, it's not surprising that the after-effects of this can spread far and wide. This often spreads to the bedroom, where it's pyjamas on and lights off before even considering getting close to our beloveds. Our stomachs are often bloated and painful, we are scarred from surgery and our backsides are often so strained that it feels as if we've been sitting on a cheese-grater rollercoaster for 15 hours solid. Not the most alluring, as you can imagine. The bottom line is always: if you feel insecure and unattractive, you don't necessarily want to take your clothes off. Try to remember that your partner probably doesn't even notice (or care) that your tum looks as if it has an entire bun factory in the oven. All of the issues you are fixated on are utter non-issues for the person who shares your bed. Intimacy and body confidence are about more than just a physical 'act'; they're about sharing everything with one another. If that involves sharing your fears and insecurities, try it. I'm sure you'll be pleasantly surprised by the response.

EXHAUSTION

It's no huge revelation that extreme fatigue is a common symptom of IBD. So when we think of bed, our first thoughts generally drift more towards snoring than sexy times. Our bodies are sleep deprived and almost constantly exhausted. We generally need more sleep than sex, and if we're not sleeping enough our libidos shut down. The general solution to this would, of course, be to ensure we get enough sleep, however that's hardly realistic in our cases – we could be asleep for 100 years and still wake up feeling as if we'd gone ten rounds with Rocky Balboa. Anaemia and iron deficiencies are also common in patients with IBD and they similarly cause an increase in these feelings of sluggishness. See your doctor regularly to ensure you are taking all of the right supplements and getting the iron infusions and/or B12 injections you sorely need.

PAIN

Last but by no means least, pain and discomfort can be major sex serial killers. When you don't feel good, your desire can take a serious hit. The last thing you want to do is consider sexual gymnastics when you can barely turn over without agonising pain. Sex should always be pleasurable, so if something is painful during intercourse, that's understandably going to cause a decrease in libido. It may initially seem mortifying, but try to talk openly with your partner about how to make things more comfortable – for both of you. Then, and only then, you'll find yourself livin' libido loco.

Bedroom gymnastics aside though, it really hadn't occurred to me just how much of a difference being diagnosed with Crohn's would make to my own relationship. There was suddenly a whole other selection box of worries for me to deliberate over. Would he want to stick around? How would I adapt if I ended up with a colostomy bag? Would I ever be physically attractive to him again? Would he or I feel differently? Would I even have the confidence to show anything more than a bare ankle to anyone, ever, again?

Yes I'm well aware this all sounds very dramatic, but these were all genuine fears and thoughts that were going through my head on a continuous mental loop after my diagnosis.

It's easy to see how difficult things can be, on both sides, in sharing a life with someone who suffers from a chronic illness. In any well-functioning relationship, both parts of a couple should always be seen as equal. This can frequently be hard to maintain when one half of a supposed partnership often finds themself in the position of playing nursemaid to the other, in the long or short term. Or in cases where one is unable to work due to chronic illness and the partner is left to take on the role of breadwinner. Financial strain is often an incredible pressure in many of even the most solid of relationships, so if the issue arises where one becomes more, or wholly, financially dependent on the other, it can cause immense strain and even potential resentment.

There is also the added burden on the patient (usually brought on through no fault of the partner I hasten to add) to revert to their normal levels of intimacy, which, after time and possibly highly intrusive surgery or merely due to the volume of symptoms suffered, may be changed indefinitely. This may in turn lead to periods of sexual abstinence, which can be a vicious circle if not discussed openly and honestly.

Understandably, these complications can all serve to put a strain on the most longstanding relationships.

Looking at things in the only way I can – from the patient's perspective – I've found all these aspects of the disease incredibly hard to adapt to. When I was unable to return work for several months after my surgery, my partner and I were forced to scrimp and save in order to make ends meet. We were struggling financially due to me having to take time off to recover and my partner taking leave to care for me as best he could. I felt tremendously guilt-ridden, as *mentally* I felt fit for work but *physically* it was completely out of the question to attempt anything that involved more exertion than making a cup of tea. (I had, however, gotten Jaffa-Cake-from-packet removal down to a fine art within mere hours of returning home.) I'd never been in the position where I wasn't earning and therefore against my will I, regrettably, became reliant on others.

Only a few months prior to my operation, my partner and I had moved into our first home together: allegedly, the most stressful thing a couple can do. We bought our house, moved in and were barely unpacked when the letter with a date for my operation swiftly popped through our shiny new letterbox. Amazingly, we didn't lose control of our faculties and fall to pieces with the strain of it all. It was almost reassuring, as we had something to focus on and work towards, and any home-related stresses we had expected didn't get the chance to come into play until I was home and in the midst of my recovery.

These tensions aside, I absolutely loathed the whole process of being 'looked after'. Certainly in the beginning. I am very fond of my own independence and find being hospitalised or bedbound incredibly uncomfortable. No amount of puffed-up pillows and daytime TV can erase the fact that you are an 'invalid'. I was in a rush to get 'back to normal'.

Crohn's takes the control away from you, as the sufferer, which can be frustrating and often surprisingly unnerving. In my case, my partner does his utmost to ensure I am tended to if I'm ever in need, but it's hard for me to feel that I'm the reason that he has to.

If I'm struggling with these occasional feelings, I often try to think of how *I* would perform were the colon in the other body. Then I feel my worries drift away, because I know that I wouldn't hesitate in doing anything and everything I could to make him well.

So I relent, as much as I can, and allow myself to be pandered too for a wee while.

Plus, there are always benefits.*

FOR YOUR EYES CROHNLY

Another area to consider for many Crohnies is how the illness affects their working relationships.

As we've discussed, Crohn's is such a complex and often baffling disease, with so many varied and wide-ranging symptoms, that it takes time, patience and effort on outsider's behalf to get to grips with everything it entails. Having an employer who takes the time to learn about your condition is a true blessing. It can mean the difference between having a comfortable working life and one where you are in constant fear of unemployment. I've been on both sides

---

* Biscuits. *Lots* of biscuits.

of that particular diseased coin, and therefore know how vital it is to be honest from the get-go and explain to your boss what affect your condition may have on your work. Even if you feel it may have a negative impact on your position, or an unfavourable reaction, nothing good ever comes of withholding the truth. Even if you feel it is your right to keep your condition to yourself, if the moment arises when you become really unwell it will take some of the heat away from constantly explaining that you are not on the brink of death.

Relationships with employers can often be tricky tightropes to walk at the best of times, let alone with a chronic illness thrown in the mix. You can't really allow yourself to become *too* friendly, as you have to remain professional and you don't ever want to feel your manager is under the impression you are using your illness as a means to avoid certain, perhaps more challenging, aspects of your job. Of course, that issue should only ever occur if you give rise to suspicion that this is something you'd be capable of doing in the first place. Certainly in my experience, most Crohn's patients have too much to concern themselves with in terms of just trying to get through the day without plotting any evil schemes to skive off from work. For me especially, sick leave = failure.

It's certainly a great expectation to assume you may have anywhere near that same level of care from an employer as you would from a loved one, but, as patients, we should certainly expect them to understand and, where possible, make certain appropriate allowances for you within the boundaries of their, and your, position.

When starting or even looking for new employment with a chronic illness, how you and the business will adapt to your illness can be a major worry. You may struggle to decide when to tell them, for fear of being turned down for a position or even pitied. My only advice there would be to ensure you are honest; it really is for the best in my experience. Never allow anyone to underestimate you. That will only happen if you allow it to.

When you have an issue such as Crohn's that often goes unseen and unspoken, one that people often struggle to grasp, it can be incredibly frustrating to find yourself in the situation whereby you have to start afresh and explain your condition to new faces from scratch. It can often feel you are constantly trying to justify why you are not only sick today, but you will STILL be sick tomorrow and the next day, and the next day, and the day after that. You get the general idea.

A previous boss of mine just didn't get it. He wanted a straightforward case of employee is ill then well – back to work as normal. When, in reality, he had me in and out of hospital with minimal information with which to furnish him.

I wasn't getting any better and had no clue when, or if, I would.

My boss after him was a revelation; she understood that if I couldn't get in contact with her straight away it was because I was in agony/on the toilet/in hospital/or all of the above.

She knew I would not, and would never, take advantage of my work due to my condition. But then she took the time to get to know me *and* my illness. This is something that requires consideration on the part of the employer and is massively appreciated by the employee. Crohn's sufferers don't expect everyone to bone up on their bowels, but when the condition affects our work it can be a huge reassurance to feel we have the confidence to talk openly to someone who is interested enough to listen.

When the time comes that a patient must change jobs, or their manager moves on, it can be a daunting prospect.

Any new relationship or position, work or otherwise (nudge, nudge, wink, wink), can be an intimidating thought. I suppose the best we can hope for as patients is to be blessed with someone understanding, who is prepared to listen and learn where necessary.

And someone who isn't too afraid of the unknown...*

TUM'S THE WORD

Relationships with family and friends can also be a tricky tightrope to walk with Crohn's Disease.

Thankfully, I find myself blessed with an incredibly supportive family and a close-knit group of friends who are always there for me to lean on (this may quite often be literally). I realise how exceptionally lucky I am to have that physical and metaphorical support and try my utmost to show them how appreciative I am of their continual, and seemingly boundless, love and backing as regularly as I can.

My friends and family hold it together incredibly well when I'm seriously ill and/or in hospital. They do their best to share funny stories of the outside world to keep

---

* Discussing our rear ends...

me up to date with the latest news/gossip, bring flowers and chocolates when I *can* eat and cuddle me silly (albeit incredibly gently).

I, in turn, will serve up Oscar-worthy performances of 'I'm fine, I really am feeling much better!' accompanied by Cheshire-cat-style smiles during these visits, then fall apart and weep a thousand self-pitying tears the minute my visitors leave the ward.

On these varied and regular instances in hospital, and there have been a good few, I've mostly felt completely and utterly alone. Regardless of the fact that during visiting hours, at the end of a phone or through the wonders of social networking, I was consistently surrounded by loved ones, I wasn't *literally* surrounded by them, and that's what I really wanted. I *needed* to be at home, amongst my loved ones and home comforts (cats). In fact, in the early days I often told little white lies to the doctors that I felt better than I actually did in order to receive a cheeky (and highly irresponsible) get-out-of-hospital-free card.

A fruitless exercise in itself, as I'd inevitably end up back in the same ward a mere few days later, shamefaced and in an even worse state than I was before. Highly 'ill'- advised I know (*now anyway*), but hospitals can often be such awfully depressing places. Especially when you have diseases related to your nether regions and are a young man/woman. The average age of the fellow patients in most of the wards I've frequented has been around 103. And that's just the nurses.

I think it's safe to say that during my numerous hospital visits to date, I've completed more word searches and crosswords than should be legally permitted in the UK and watched elderly ladies remove their false teeth more often than I've brushed my own in my entire lifetime. If there was a hospital-stay equivalent of air miles I'd be well on my way to Barbados.

Family wise, my mother in particular has been affected a great deal by my illness. She worries about me constantly; when I preach that it's really not necessary, as I'm big enough and certainly ugly enough to worry for both of us, it always falls entirely on deaf ears. One of my brothers is also chronically unwell and she has said she feels somehow responsible. She reasons that as we are both created of her and my dad's genes, it stands to reason that she is to blame in some way. This is irrespective of my continued protestations otherwise.

Crohn's is not hereditary and there is absolutely no history of it in my immediate family history. Even if it were, it wouldn't be her or my father's 'fault' – they would never wish this on any of their children to begin with, and I have never even given 'blaming' them a first, let alone second, thought. It really is irrelevant to me how I ended up with Crohn's. Finding out how it came to pass that my bowels should have ended up in the diseased state they are in won't change a thing. It certainly may have helped in diagnosing my condition. If there *had* been a family member who had suffered from the same illness, or something similar, I would've at the very least known what the hell it was. It would've also been a handy 'disease template' to work from in attempting to uncover what was going on inside. Nevertheless, thankfully and wonderfully, the majority of my loved ones are relatively healthy.

My mother feels that she should be the one who is ill. She hates having two of her three children suffer from conditions they will likely have to endure for the rest of their lives.

Endurance is, coincidentally, a word I associate with Crohn's quite regularly. Living day by day with a chronic illness feels very much like a test of mental and physical stamina. An endurance test with no first, second or third prizes, no popping of bottles of champagne or neck-breaking golden medals at the end of it. Not even so much as a chocolate medal, because technically there is no end – it's incurable. That means this particular test of endurance will go on and on until your light inevitably fades out.

I often find myself withholding certain nuggets of health-related information from my darling mum, until completely necessary at least, as I know she worries to the point of making *herself* ill. It's another consideration to be weighed up, as much as I adore her, as the last thing we would want (or need) is for my mum and me to find ourselves stuck next to one another on a hospital ward. For a start she is SO much better at crosswords than me, and I don't need that level of competition when I'm already feeling like death.

My wonderful mum gets anxious when I don't finish a meal, when I spend too long in the bathroom or when I complain of the tiniest of tummy twinges. If she sees me grimace in pain – something I tend to do without even being aware of it – she falls into a panic.

In the beginning I would often catch her looking at me as though I were almost made of glass and the slightest wrong movement would cause me to shatter into a million pieces all over her freshly hoovered carpet. Who am I kidding? That still happens and probably always will.

Not being a mother myself, I can't begin to imagine how distressing it must be when your child is poorly, no matter what age they are. So I do my absolute utmost to bear that in mind when my mum gets stressed over my own ill health. I try to explain that her constant concern for me is much appreciated, truly, but knowing that she is worried doesn't serve to ease my pain – in fact it often only makes me uptight and causes stress that serves to exacerbate my symptoms. Although all the while I know these complaints are futile, as it's in her make-up to be apprehensive, and no amount of sweet-talking or telling offs from me will make one iota of difference.

I suppose because all these visible symptoms are so commonplace to me now, it's always slightly irksome when people comment or even get anxious about them. I can't explain *why* exactly, but it just tends to feel that they are getting worked up over nothing. That's not in any way a bad thing, it's a wonderful feeling to know people care for you and your well-being, it can just get a little overwhelming at times.

Friends and family can also often get more frustrated than the patient over a doctor's actions.

YOU are their wife/daughter/friend/mother, therefore it's ONLY FAIR and RIGHT and JUST that YOU should be right at the top of their priority list!

As a patient, however, you quickly become (disappointingly) only too well aware that YOUR doctor has OTHER sick people to see and that regrettably you are just another ill person in a long day filled with ill people.

But those people who love you understandably feel you should be considered so much more. Because to them, just like Diana Ross was to Marvin Gaye, you *are* everything. They feel you should be, at the very least, welcomed into the doctor's office with open arms after gracefully wafting along a red carpet, while the existing patient exits the room clutching their prescription via a trapdoor. It's only right! And fair! And just!

I do understand of course that seeing a loved one suffer is beyond awful. I've been on the other side of the hospital bed myself, staring expectantly at someone I love when they've been decidedly under the weather. Sitting alongside them, and feeling all those same mixed-up feelings that go along with it: pity, sadness, empathy and hope. Dry mouthed and struggling at the sheer helplessness of seemingly never being able to find the right healing words to say. Racking your brain to come up with the latest gossip, funny story or OH MY GOD THE CAT DID THEEEEE CUTEST THING that might make your patient smile. That almost overwhelming urge to pick up your beloved like Richard Gere in *An Officer and a Gentleman* and gracefully carry them aloft out of the ward towards freedom and decent tea and biscuits. All 100 per cent natural feelings.

So I'm told.

ICE CREAM CROHN'S

The difficulty I often find in coping with Crohn's is trying to separate how I feel with how it must feel to be on the outside of this disease.

What must it be like to be friends with someone with a chronic illness, for example?

In my case, my close friends have been incredibly understanding and tolerant of my illness. That may sound strange, but it's not easy learning your BFF is going to be poorly FO' EVA. Let's face it, it's not 'fun' having Crohn's. It can stop you doing things (e.g. activities), or people (e.g. intercourse!) you love. It can also keep you from spending time with those you normally would. Friends of patients with a chronic illness unfortunately have to learn to become flexible in order to remain in your life.

Being diagnosed with an incurable illness and one that can be so...unpleasant...can serve as a surprisingly useful tool for weeding out anything 'stale' amongst your intimate circle. Any 'dead wood' within your friendships will start to fall by the wayside and the people you can rely on will start to shine through.

Those individuals in your life who genuinely WANT to know how you are will become decidedly more apparent and those who ask after you just for the sake of it, or because they feel they have to in order to maintain a polite façade, will become distinctly more aggravating.

Having the disease has helped me to see clearly who I can truly rely on in my time of need. This wasn't something that I'd rated particularly highly on the

Friendship Scale until I was eventually diagnosed. Friends who genuinely care for you and for your well-being will happily reschedule plans, content in the knowledge that the main consideration is that you are ok.

My bosom buddies don't ever complain and gripe about having been stood up; without having to think about it they will ask how I am and if there's anything they can do to ease my suffering.

True friends will come to you if you are too unwell or physically unable to get to them. They will laugh along with you at the antics of your idiotic body, and in turn give you full access to their sizeable shoulders if those moments when you need to have a cry about things arise. They will take the time to learn exactly what your condition entails and, more importantly, they will try to understand it.

Crohn's patients can, in the long or short term, find themselves becoming much less sociable than perhaps they once were. The symptoms of the illness can be so unsavoury that the last thing you feel like doing is hitting the dance floor and boogying till dawn. Saturday Night Fever has never felt so apt.

Eating habits and alcohol intake may have to adapt to suit the disease, which can in turn serve to change some previously best-laid plans. The 'invisibility' of the condition means communication truly is the key aspect to remember in dealing with loved ones. Extreme fatigue, low self-esteem and the more gruesome internal indicators can all go unnoticed to the untrained eye, so it's vital the patient expresses how they are feeling inside to allow friends to make inroads in beginning to understand.

At our worst we almost constantly feel like throwing up or rushing to the toilet or are in often excruciating pain. That's incredibly hard to comprehend when you can't see or feel it happening.

It's also easy to say you *know* what someone with Crohn's is going through, but you don't. Not *really*. Not unless you have been with them when they are at rock bottom and certainly not just when they are well. Fairweather friends are little to no use to Crohn's patients, as we often require an umbrella more than sunglasses. Snow shoes over sun lotion. You get the general idea. For us the forecast can be so frustratingly changeable that if you're coming along for the ride you have to come prepared for every eventuality.

This requires dedication and perseverance that, unfortunately, some people often lack.

Friendship for me (disease aside for just a moment) should be based on shared interests, honesty and laughter. *LOTS of laughter.* It genuinely is one of the best medicines. And absolutely FREE!!

You should be able to talk to a friend about anything that's on your mind without fear of judgement or anxiety that what you are saying may be misconstrued in any way. A good friend should be able to cheer you up, and hold you up during the bad times (in my case often physically as well as metaphorically).

So why should those friendship priorities change if one half of the relationship becomes sick and the other half is still fit as a fiddle?

Many fellow Crohn's sufferers I've spoken to on this subject have commented that shortly after their diagnosis they've found, much to their dismay, that many of their friends have become distant. Or that they've openly admitted they've had difficulty in adapting to having a 'sick' friend. Sometimes, being labelled as sickly through no fault of our own can be infuriating. Being offered the sympathy card once too often can also put a massive strain on the dynamics of any friendship, regardless of how longstanding it may be.

Many new patients find themselves withdrawing from friendships because they don't want to be considered a burden or simply because they don't want to talk about their illness AGAIN, especially when in the midst of a flare-up. This can push those closest away at times, but it may every so often show the patient who's prepared to stick around. It all depends on the type of person, I suppose.

Many friends can find it hard to avoid the diseased elephant in the room and conversations can dry up when only one is making an effort, in turn making both parties feel increasingly uncomfortable. Unfortunate, but easily avoided if both patient and pal take a minute to talk openly and don't expect too much from one another.

From my own experiences, I believe that you often don't truly know or appreciate someone until these times of crisis occur. It quickly becomes blatantly, and often painfully, clear who will stick around. These are generally the people in your life who would never so much as consider the alternative.

I'm incredibly thankful for the friends I've gained over the years. It can become increasingly difficult the older you get to make any new friends that 'stick'. I have a few precious, lifelong friends, and I've been lucky enough to gather some new ones over the years. Friends who I know will now always play a big part in the melodrama that is my life. They might even get a special mention in the credits.

CROHNLY LOVE

Although it's very important as a friend of a Crohnie to be prepared for all the ups and downs you will inevitably encounter along the way, it's also vital to remember the one who is suffering too.

What is the role of the patient in this incredibly important friendship scenario?

For myself, in the beginning I felt that for no reason other than because *I* was the sickly one, the 'injured party' so to speak, *I* should be the one my friends made all the allowances for. *They* should be there for *me* whenever I needed them, actively and forcefully telling me everything will be fine.

Little did I realise quite how much my diagnosis was also affecting them.

A few of my treasured friends, knowing little of the condition following my initial diagnosis, came to their own conclusions about what would happen to me in the coming weeks and months. Many thought that Crohn's was a psycho killer (Qu'est-ce que c'est?) and that my diagnosis was that of a terminal illness. A lot of people wrongly assume this is the case when first hearing the word 'incurable'. It's understandable to a certain extent and must've been a terrifying time for them too. One of my closest friends told me she wished I'd had something 'trifling' like IBS or that she could swap places with me. She was often heartbroken seeing me in hospital but visited me regularly and brought flowers and, more importantly, hopeful smiles with her. That's all anyone can do really – try to help you see things more positively. Even on the occasions when perhaps they struggle to see the light at the end of your colon too.

As the patient in question it's important to value yourself, even when you probably feel worthless. Try to remember at all times that you are someone they love and that they hate to see you in any form of pain and suffering.

As with any form of relationship, it's vital you attempt to see situations from their point of view. Think about how you would feel were it *them* staring weakly back at *you* from a hospital bed. Although you are perhaps the invalid, those around you still need a little support too. You can't be expected to be all things to all people, just allow yourself to be honest with your loved ones and don't feel you have to lie in any way, or sugar coat things purely for their benefit. Those who truly care will worry about you regardless, so as the patient allow that where you can, but don't let them wallow. It won't aid your mental health or their wee hearts.

If you happen to be the one paying a visit to your poorly pal and all you can do is keep them up to date with what's happening in the outside world, then simply do that. Believe me when I say that actions that you may consider only tiny can be gargantuan to the patient concerned.

As a seasoned professional in tormenting myself that I'll lose everyone I love due to my horrid disease… I feel I'm quite the authority. So here are my TOP TIPS for you and your loved ones in maintaining positive relationships whilst living with a chronic illness:

1. HAVE A LITTLE PATIENCE

Don't rush your friend into opening up to you about their illness. It can often take a very long time before patients are able to admit to themselves what's happening to their bodies, let alone discuss it with anyone on the outside. It can take time to process the news and the inevitable information overload they are met with, particularly on diagnosis. Often, friends are left in the dark during this stretch. Have faith and perseverance that it will pass and that you can share more, if not everything, in good time. All the patient needs from you in the first instance is to let them know you will be there waiting when they are good and ready to open up. They've probably done enough 'opening up' of their more intimate cavities to last a good few months at the minute.

2. REIN IN THE SYMPATHY

If at all feasible, try to go easy on the feeling-sorry-for-patients patter. As Crohn's sufferers we do like being given a little bit of an allowance now and then and, yes, occasionally we do tend to enjoy wallowing in self-pity, but please do not encourage that behaviour. Don't give it big licks with the apologetic glances and sympathetic head tilts. We get more than enough of that from doctors and nurses. We never want to feel that we have somehow changed in your eyes or that you feel let down on our behalf. That's just the absolute WORST from people you love. There's a pity party in our pants 24 hours a day; we don't need you to join in too.

3. THERE WILL BE BOWELS

We are going to talk about what's coming out of our backside from time to time. If you can't deal with that you'll now regrettably have to learn how. It's an unfortunate part of our lives and, as very bestest buddies, our social lives may be disrupted by it at times too. We have had to learn so much about our bottoms it hurts (quite often literally). We aren't by any manner of means asking you to do the same, just to try to be patient and if necessary grit your teeth occasionally if you have to hear about our rears and what they've been up to.

Besides, we have to tolerate your stories about how Tom/Dick/Harry has stood you up AGAIN; the least you can do is take part in discussing my stool leaving *me* from time to time (albeit less regularly).

4. EXCLUSION CROHN

From time to time we may begin to feel disheartened and this can make itself more visibly known in the way we spend our time. Crohn's can often contribute greatly to the fear of going out in public in case we have an 'accident' or throw up or both. Together.

It can be an intimidating prospect, and the more you start to focus on these fears the more withdrawn you can become. It can happen before you even realise it. At times like these it is often vital that friends and loved ones try to help break that cycle. Even if it's something as simple as making sure they check in with you if you ever go MIA. If you have any worries that your loved one may be on a downward spiral then try to act quickly and subtly. Don't betray their trust by rushing with your fears to their families (that may just inflame the situation); take the first step in voicing your fears and see where that leads. Keep a close eye on them and keep in touch as regularly as you can to see how things are progressing for them.

It's also important to maintain a good balance with your friend and not to push too hard. The patient may have hang-ups about issues that seem paltry and unimportant to you, such as using toilets elsewhere or the panic of establishing where the lavatory is situated when visiting a new place – bear in mind these may sound trivial to you but are real worries and potential panics for a Crohnie.

5. CROHNLY TIME WILL TELL

Don't push. This may seem to be a contradiction to point number four, but by 'pushing' I refer to attempts to force us into doing certain things or going to places we went before. Bear in mind the changes to our bodies we are currently dealing with and, often more importantly, our mental state. Try to think about how a situation or suggestion would affect us NOW, not pre-Crohn's. Just ask gently but don't get offended if we aren't up to whatever you propose, whatever it may be and however small an issue *you* may think it is. Things may not have changed too much as far as friends and family are concerned but we can suddenly feel as if we are an oddity in a world that seems to have moved on without us. A massive lifestyle change has taken place for us as patients and we have to take time to adapt to that. Try not to get annoyed if we can't party as hard as we used to. We may get there eventually, albeit with more toilet breaks…

6. A MIND OF MY CROHN

Get smart. It's imperative as someone who loves a Crohnie to learn all you can about their condition. We certainly aren't asking you to swot up and gain a borderline medical degree (although that would be GREAT), but it helps massively to allow you to understand what we are going through. And even what may lie ahead. This is especially important if your friend happens to be struggling to understand the condition. Help them learn and it will aid you both. Knowing a bit of background about the facts and figures in living with Crohn's can also help both parties keep track of how the disease may affect your relationship, now and in the future. The patient starts to notice the signs they are going downhill pretty quickly, so as someone who spends a lot of time with them it's something you will logically start to recognise too. That's the theory anyway.

7. CROHNLY YOU

Lack of intimacy isn't a lack of love. Intimacy can be hard to maintain with Crohn's, as the illness tends to affect our 'downstairs' areas. When you are back and forth from the toilet every five minutes, vomiting, sweating and feeling like death, somewhat understandably, any closeness with another person is about the furthest thing from your mind. Unless you find having your fevered brow mopped particularly sensual. This can be incredibly hard for a partner or a close friend to adapt to because they aren't feeling what you feel and don't have the same distractions to concern themselves that you do. It's important to explain why you aren't feeling particularly attractive or perhaps 'in the mood' – but whatever you do don't leave your partner in the dark; if they love you they will understand. But only if *you* let them.

8. GET CREATIVE

This suggestion can apply in friendship, family or romantic situations. Don't always assume our illness will limit everything. We are not made primarily of porcelain; we just tend to find ourselves getting more intimate with it than most a lot of the time. In some cases the condition we suffer from will undoubtedly limit our ability to do certain things, but it's important to do your best to get your thinking cap on and come up with alternative activities or ways to resolve issues so that we don't feel left out or isolated. We absolutely do not want to ruin plans for others, and definitely don't intend to, but we can't always see a solution to certain problems when we feel at our worst. There will always be a practical resolution if you think hard enough. If we can't go out then come to us. With wine obviously – always bring wine. If we can't do it doggy style because my rear is in uproar then find another position. Again, always bring wine. (Sorry Dad.)

9. TELL ME ABOUT YOUR COLD

Another common issue many loved ones of Crohn's sufferers encounter is falling under the misguided assumption that they are somehow not permitted to be 'sick' themselves because sufferers have an incurable illness – that even the mere mention of it will somehow offend our delicate sensibilities. Obviously, the idea of a life not blighted by as much as a head cold is ridiculous (and sadly practically impossible), but I can see why it arises. It's a very common misconception amongst my friends in particular, who tend to fall into discussion of their sickly symptoms then vaguely panic and offset it with something along the lines of: 'It's obviously nothing compared to what you are going through though...'

They feel that it will seem selfish to complain about something trivial when we are suffering and poorly 365 days of the year. But it's not. Not unless you do it ALL THE TIME, obviously. Just as your loved ones want to be kept up to date with your health, we too want to be informed if someone we care for is feeling under the weather. We aren't going to jump down your throat if you tell us you have a cold. Unless it's just after we've come round from a triple bypass...then it's a little inappropriate.

I naturally want to know about anything – good or bad – that's happening to my friend! Besides, our medical knowledge is usually second to none…

10. I AM STILL ME

Finally, the main problem newly diagnosed patients seem to experience is a pressure to discuss their new-fangled illness with others. For me, once the novelty/shock of the diagnosis wore off and we all tried to go about our daily lives, some friends admitted they found it increasingly hard to separate 'Sick Kath' from just plain old 'Kath'. Friends can quickly become uncomfortable and feel they have to mention the disease at all times or we'll somehow be offended. As if we will feel that if it's not discussed they'll have temporarily forgotten or that they aren't putting us and our health first. Or, worse, if you don't mention it we'll somehow fall apart. Here's a potential revelation though: *we don't actually want to talk about Crohn's all day every day.* We want to attempt to carry on with our lives as normally as is achievable, and we want you to treat us in exactly the same way you always have. *Not* with kid gloves.

Crohn's can certainly be life changing, but you can never allow it to alter every aspect of your life. As someone who cares about us, it's vital you do your utmost to ensure we never stop chanting that mantra.

5

FINISH

THE PHILOSOPHER'S CROHN

Friday 28 January 2011
'Managed a shower today (with the help of the nurse). Little victories! That Les Dawson-looking woman in the ward opposite is going to feel my wrath if she doesn't cease the "me me me" patter IMMEDIATELY.'

Tuesday 1 February 2011
'He came to pick me up to take me home, he came into the ward dancing!'

YOU DON'T CROHN ME

There's unfortunately no denying Crohn's Disease can play havoc with your head as well as your insides. I've found that the biggest challenge to be faced in living with Crohn's is ensuring it doesn't get its vice-like grip on your mental health, as well as your physical health.

Personally, incurable disease considered, I don't feel that the life I have is a particularly hard one.

I have a full-time job, a mortgage, a man I adore and an amazing family and bunch of friends whom I love unconditionally. I don't have much money as such, but I have just enough to get the bills paid and have a little left over for some fun/cat outfits/jars of Nutella. I'd say I have a pretty good social life and hobbies, and I am blessed with people around me who make me laugh until my sides ache. I have cats that are the feline apples of my eye and I get to pet them anytime I like, whether THEY like it or not.

So with all that unbridled joy in my life, why do I sometimes feel so unbearably low that I could fill a loch with my own salty tears?

There is a colloquial saying in my home country of Scotland that goes: 'Well at least you have your health!'

I think this phrase is perhaps designed to instil hope and encouragement in its recipient. The theory being that whatever happens, however bad things have become, however utterly hopeless you may feel in this moment, at least you're not dead!

Over the years, for me that particular saying has gone from being one that I used to hear intermittently uttered by the over-eighties of my local area – reciting this banal phrase, parrot-like at the end of every conversation – to realising as I got older that it was utterly pointless and redundant. Eventually, finding its mere utterance such an unbearable cliché, I considered it almost laughable. I find just the sheer expression of it tends to come out peppered with unnecessary bitterness.

The truth is, grannies of Scotland and beyond, I *don't* have my health.

I have an incredibly unpleasant and incurable illness, which I will most likely have until the day I meet that great David Bowie in the sky.

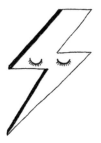

The vast majority of my twenties have been spent under a murky cloud of illness. This simple fact isn't going to change; those are my resounding memories of that frisky decade. I fully intend to ensure, to the very best of my ability, that my thirties, forties and beyond are so very much better. But, as with any plans for the future, my disease will almost certainly have the final say in this.

Every day I am abundantly aware that I have Crohn's. It's a fact that's simply impossible to avoid.

I wake up and go to bed at night having felt it/thought about it/been irritated by it (or all of the above and maybe more). But on occasional days, I KNOW I have Crohn's. It hits me like a bolt from the blue and I find myself absolutely floored by it. These moments usually come after, or during, a bad flare-up. But sometimes they are wholly unexpected. Often, the reminder I am genuinely not ever 'getting better' and that repeating realisation are almost too much to bear. I become entirely overwhelmed.

I can feel as if I am on the outside looking in on myself, and in that exact moment I feel utterly hopeless.

As I slowly adapt to my disease more and more with each passing flare-up and symptom, these 'blue' days are, thankfully, few and far between. The majority of the time, I have a very positive outlook on my life and my disease. I'm well aware that my condition won't ever go away, and I try to make the best of what is, literally, a shit situation. That isn't at all easy at times, but it's unquestionably essential.

In those certain moments when I'm feeling low about my illness, I'm LOW.

I'm the limbo champion of the world.

I'm a broken paving slab, downtrodden into the dirt after a particularly heavy Scottish rainfall.

I'm a classic 1977 David Bowie album.

You get the general idea.

It's a position that I find incredibly difficult to climb out of. These feelings of despair and sheer misery are challenging enough to deal with on their own, but they are compounded by my own pummelling frustration at myself. Why are you suddenly getting upset about this now?! You've had it for years! Get a grip of yourself! ETC. *To infinity.*

It's this mental, vicious circle that can seem almost unbearably hard to break. This is the aspect of Crohn's Disease and many other chronic illnesses that, for the most part, goes unspoken.

Not by me. I am infuriated by, but not in the slightest bit ashamed of, these feelings. That doesn't mean to say that they don't antagonise and frustrate me, because they do, incredibly so.

But unlike Crohn's itself they are always temporary. These occasional and erratic blue moods are a part of my illness and therefore a part of my life and, like the Terminator himself, they will be back.

I have accepted my condition, but I know it will hit me brick-in-the-face hard again from time to time. That's undoubtedly not something I look forward to, but I don't intend to spend my entire existence waiting for it either. I live my life to the fullest and to the best of my ability when I have the physical and mental capacity to do so. I try not to be too hard on myself when I don't.

Please follow my lead and never allow yourself to be anything less than honest with yourself, and the people who love you. Your feelings are not, and never will be, your failings.

CROHN FISHING

Let's face it: Crohn's is an endurance test. A constant challenge that cannot be overcome, just controlled and contained. As we've mentioned, you can change the way you look at it, but what about the way *it* makes *you* look?

Over the past few years I'm pleasantly surprised to find that I've started to notice a shift in my attitude towards both my disease and my body.

I've become much less hung up on how I look and definitely less interested in how I appear to others.

A life-changing illness tends to sort the wheat from the chaff in terms of priorities.

This former preoccupation with my personal appearance seems to have been a consistently long-running theme throughout my teens, following on obstreperously into my twenties. A common scenario for most young women, it would appear. It's certainly a frame of mind I'm finally glad to be shaking off.

Most of my youth, up to the age of around 16, was spent looking (and behaving) distinctly like a tomboy. I'd spend chunks of my days absentmindedly wondering if I'd ever encounter those mythical possessions known as 'breasts' on my *own* body. Training bras just weren't cutting it for me anymore. I knew I was faking it. Boys could tell. What was I in 'training' for anyway? And how much training did I have to endure exactly – whatever it was I'd excelled in it by now, yet still, NOTHING!

I was in equal measure terrified of those bulbous appendages and utterly desperate to covet them. Thankfully, this desperation didn't stretch to making any visual 'modifications' to my ironing-board chest such as firing socks down my jumper or padding out my training bra with newspaper; instead I attempted to wait patiently and resigned myself to the fact I'd be unappealing to the opposite sex until the day they arrived.

I didn't realise at the time that I actually wasn't entirely unappealing to the opposite sex. I must have given them very little credit. I did have 'boy-*friends*', which is a phrase I seemed to take literally – emphasis on the 'friend'. Blossoming boy-men did begin to take an interest in me because I was allegedly funny and not borderline brain-dead, but I never at any point thought these interests were of the 'let's go behind the bike sheds' variety. I just assumed they wanted to hear me do funny voices or more daft impressions of the teachers. Mrs Jenkins was my specialty, since you ask.

Anyway, time passed and I grew and grew... And grew... And all hell broke loose. I won't elaborate, for my dad's sake, and I'll have to look him in the eye.

Over time (which always seems endless when you are a teenager), I became more paranoid about how I looked. I told myself I didn't care, because it was *such a girly cliché*, but I did. I was borderline obsessed with my stomach – it was always bloated and sore – and although I was absolutely stick-insect thin I always felt 'fat'. I wasn't.

Don't get me wrong, I by no means had any form of eating disorder, and I certainly never let these preadolescent feelings get in the way of my day-to-day life. I ate, but again only wee bits here and there – the smallest of portions. I'd feel absolutely starving, only manage a few mouthfuls and swiftly be full. Not just 'satisfied' but full up to the point of feeling sick and bloated after every single meal. This was my life though; I hadn't known anything else so why would I complain? Why would I suspect my body worked any differently to anyone else's? And why, oh why, couldn't I fit into those flares (yes, flares, I should've been born in the seventies) one minute then have them fall down from my bony hips *in public* the next?

These bloated and crampy pains after eating were a chore in my youth. Working, studying and doing funny voices all started to take their toll on my delicate stomach and frail Bambi-esque frame. As I matured and stepped into the world of work, these issues became a little more apparent. Friends and colleagues would tell me they worried I that seemingly ate so little and even felt guilty that they could demolish a plate of food in half the time I could finish a couple of forkfuls. But again I really didn't think anything of it; I just assumed I had a small appetite or possibly a small stomach?

I felt fat, as my stomach ballooned mere moments after eating and drinking, and this often caused repeated internal tantrums; there was no point in making an effort to look good when I felt as if I was a beached whale. I looked milk-bottle white the majority of the time and was always icy cold to the touch.

Thank the Lord Bowie in heaven that those boys remembered their portable heaters when we went to the bike sheds (JOKING, DAD).

These issues with my appetite and badly behaved bowels escalated until, inevitably, I was seriously ill.

Eventually (as I may have mentioned perhaps more than is entirely necessary), I saw a few hundred doctors and nurses and was finally diagnosed with Crohn's Disease at the ripe old age of 27.

I've had one operation, at the time of writing, and multiple shall we say unpalatable treatments. I'll undoubtedly be on medication of some form or another for the rest of my days and hospital visits and/or stays will be a thing of my future.

That's ok. It really is.

I only mention it in the hope it serves to help other people understand just quite how much the effects of a long-term illness, various drugs, persistent and intrusive medical procedures and surgery can have on your physical appearance. And in turn, how these changes to the inside of your body can really affect the way you see yourself on the outside. If you had no issues with the way the world saw you pre-Crohn's, you may find this particular outlook turned on its head not long afterwards.

When I see photos of myself at my 'unhealthiest', which are happily scarce thanks to that massive 'accidental' bonfire, I feel very saddened at just how noticeably and awfully unwell I looked. Looking back, I also feel frustrated at the knowledge that this was a situation I had absolutely no control over. No amount of make-up can disguise the fact that your body is killing you from the inside out.

I know I certainly don't want to be back in that same poorly position again, but I'm also well aware that I don't really have any say in the matter. I was in unbearable agony, doubled up like I was vainly attempting to recreate the foetal position, pale, lifeless and so thin I was dangerously underweight. Not a place I particularly want to revisit anytime soon.

But now, as I hurtle on with my future, my disease along for the ride like some unsightly appendage, I am looking to the months and years ahead with hope and a renewed sense of self. I understand that may sound a little pretentious. What I mean is that I like who I have become, diseased or not. I know my body's enforced limitations and I have accepted them. I know my figure will never be conventionally 'perfect'. Whatever that may mean in this day and age. My particular organisation of bones, flesh and organs is highly changeable, bloated, pale and scarred. But it's *mine*, and it's the only one I'll ever have. It's thus far proven itself to be a tough piece of kit and I'm proud of what I've endured and what I'm sure I will continue to endure in the years to come. You reading this: you should be too.

There are more people who think you are beautiful than you know. Embrace your illness – it's another challenge you can overcome.

Oh and for the record, I did end up with those mythical breasts, and they are quite exquisite if I do say so myself.

INTO THE DANGER CROHN

Whatever your walk of life, being diagnosed with Crohn's Disease is a life-changing event. It's terrifying and difficult and, as we've mentioned previously, a huge challenge to adapt to.

Making a conscious decision to accept your changing body and, more importantly, the changes the disease will have on your life is excellent in theory, however putting it into practice is quite another issue. It takes tremendous time, patience and, most importantly, willpower. It's important not to push yourself too soon, to allow yourself the time you need to adapt and not to allow anyone or anything to put unnecessary pressure on your state of mind. How long you may need is really down to you and possibly the severity of your diagnosis. It's a life-changing illness, often in both slight and unquestionably massive ways.

However, I feel 'life changing' can be seen as both a negative and positive. Every negative effect of the illness on your life, and of many others around you, can, thankfully, be countered with a positive one. That is if you really look hard enough for the constructive ones.

It can, understandably, be tremendously intimidating to think that there is something in your life you can't control. Especially if you are a borderline control freak like myself.

You may *think* you are in charge of your own destiny, but Crohn's regularly serves to remind you that you aren't even in charge of your own *bowels* half the time. Quite humbling at times and often totally hilarious. The idea that my body makes choices for me and my head has nothing to do with it utterly floors me. Often, literally.

Bear in mind that although it's frequently a colossal challenge to maintain a sense of humour where Crohn's is concerned, it's also VITAL. In my opinion, it allows you to seize a bit of the control back. Your body may play tricks on you, but why allow yourself to lose your dignity when you can laugh instead at the sheer ridiculousness of the situations you find yourself in? It tends to make these moments a hell of a lot easier to get over and move on from. It also gifts you some amusing anecdotes for those potentially difficult icebreaker situations.

Just be careful when you use them – FYI, they are (usually) inappropriate at funerals and weddings.

Aside from the often more obviously grisly symptoms, I find it's when Crohn's starts interfering in my personal life that things can really take a turn for the worse. It gets increasingly difficult and can, at times, be justly depressing when you find your world being turned upside down simply because your stomach has decided to do somersaults elaborate enough to qualify for the World Gymnastic Championships.

Crohn's can turn up to your party uninvited and cause complete havoc, leaving your insides in uproar and you to clean up the mess. So very RUDE.

Let's now take a look at these oft-referred to as 'life-changing' aspects of the illness in a little more detail. I hope this serves to show you, dear reader, there can be positives to the condition as well as negatives. Here's another tried-and-tested top ten…

1. CROHNA LISA: STRUGGLING WITH CONFIDENCE AND SELF-ESTEEM

Many patients feel that they lose confidence in their struggle to adapt to the illness. They feel somehow less of a person, literally so in cases of having had resection surgery. This can manifest itself in many ways. People can become quiet and introverted or even isolated and suffer from depression. Patients who have possibly suffered from any of these traits and illnesses before may, sadly, find they now have much more severe cases.

For me personally, this has been a difficult challenge to overcome. I can't say I'm entirely there yet, but I'm definitely well on my way.

After my surgery, I was ashamed and almost afraid of my own body. I hated my scar and the fact that it would forever be a seemingly nasty slant on my previously untarnished blank canvas. I couldn't bear even to look at myself for a good few weeks. I peeked only when entirely necessary – cleaning, making sure my wound was healing ok or when the surgeon was checking me over.

Now, a few years down the line, I realise that this blip on the bodily horizon is a part of me. Like those little worry wobbles you get on your forehead or the laughter lines around your eyes as you get older. It serves as a part of my 'body-map', showing me the routes and journeys my body has taken across my lifetime. If anyone asks about it I can tell them how I struggle with a chronic illness, and this was the moment I beat it. If only for a few months, I won.

Or, I can lie and terrify youngsters with that run in I had with a shark.

Crohn's sufferers are strong and beautiful. Maybe it doesn't always feel that way, but as long as we try to remember it we'll be on the right track of our maps.

2. CROHNLY THE STRONG: SCALING BACK PARTS OF YOUR LIFE

This can also be a problematic and often arduous task, especially for a newly diagnosed Crohnie. Sufferers who were perhaps once the life and soul of every party can suddenly find themselves forced to turn down invitations or leave events early due to ill health. This is something that unfortunately can't be helped, and the key is learning to cater to what your body can now handle – weighing up what you want with what you can do. This has been a tough challenge for me. I absolutely hate having to cancel plans and frequently feel I am letting down my friends and loved ones at every turn. Often, no matter how understanding and patient they are, it's something you, as the 'sick' one, can't seem to shake off mentally.

The unpredictability of the disease also means that often in the midst of a night out, or event, you can become ill and be forced to leave. You may find yourself occupying the bathroom for longer than is considered socially acceptable.

This also applies in the work environment. Often, patients find it a huge challenge to return to work after a hospital stay, surgery or a bad flare-up. Solutions may involve lessening your workload, which in many cases is not physically or financially viable.

3. CROHNLY A MATTER OF TIME: CHANGED PERSPECTIVE ON LIFE

Having this disease and making all the sacrifices and adaptations that come with it can also allow the patient a rare opportunity to see things a little more clearly. Are you in the wrong line of work? Are you as happy as you should or could be in your relationship? Are your friends truly there for you in your time of need in the same way you are for them?

The answer to all these questions may be a rousing 'yes', which is *wonderful*. But if it's a no, to one or all three, then it may be the time to get some insight into what's worth hanging on to.

You may think this is a pretty mammoth task to be taking on alongside a chronic illness, but for me it's been a gradual process and something that has happened pretty much entirely of its own accord. The way I started to view my friends and family changed. Where my parents, partner, close family and friends were concerned I felt immense love and terror at the thought of losing them all at once. Becoming ill made me acutely more aware not to take anyone I love for granted and cherishing the times we have together. The way people reacted to my illness, or those moments when I needed a shoulder to lean on, also became glaringly obvious. When I realised some were backing off, or visibly uncomfortable in discussing my situation, I had absolutely no qualms in keeping my distance, as it was now so apparent these people were not going to be in it for the long haul. And that's ok. It's a little sad, and can be incredibly disappointing, especially when someone has been a large part of your life to date. But when you are at your lowest and you feel worthless, you begin to realise how truly important it is to be loved and to hang on for dear life to those who are continually standing by your side.

4. DON'T KNOW WHAT YOU'VE GOT 'TIL IT'S CROHN: REALISE YOU ARE NOT ALONE

This is so very important in adapting to the illness. It's vital you remember that there is always someone out there who is going through the same thing that you are. Although this may perhaps sound heartless – obviously only a sadist or complete bastard would feel good knowing other people are suffering – but it's more about taking comfort in the knowledge that you are not the only one feeling the way you feel. If you were, you would end up feeling extremely stranded and utterly isolated. Like one lonely (diseased) coconut on an uninhabited desert island.

It's vital to know there are others out there who feel what you feel. This helps, not just in confirming you are not alone in your struggle, but also in being a marvellous way to find out more about the disease. Doctors obviously know their stuff when it comes to the medical ins and outs, but true experience and insight into what it's like *to live with* Crohn's Disease can only come from a fellow sufferer. Making new Crohnie friends has helped me tenfold in learning about my illness and given me invaluable hints and tips to combat all aspects of coping with it. It's also wonderful to have a virtual or physical support network around you, like a massive safety blanket there whenever you need it.

5. THE ONE AND CROHNLY: YOU'LL NEVER BE 'NORMAL'

Whatever, that word means. No one is 'normal' because, thankfully, such a person doesn't exist. Everyone is unique and wonderful in their own way. Idiots and my nemesis being the main exceptions to that rule. This idea of 'fitting in' can, unfortunately, transcend our childhood and school days and follow us awkwardly into our later life. We all spend the majority of our youth striving for acceptance from our peers, a lot of the time from people we don't even like very much ourselves. We are a funny lot, aren't we?

Having a disease like Crohn's takes you 'out of the norm'. Your body isn't functioning normally, so how can you be expected to? Your insides are *attacking* themselves – it's not *normal*. I try to allow myself to talk openly about my illness so as not to feel ashamed or as though I am hiding anything for fear of being labelled 'abnormal'.

The way in which you handle your disease really does have a bearing on this. You can bitch and whine about how hard done by you are and how awful life is, but if you start to give in to your illness you may find yourself on a slippery and miserable slope. Many who follow this dangerous path find themselves in an unpleasant position where they are labelled by their illness.

I, undoubtedly, don't want people to recoil in fear at the mere mention of my bowels but I do want them to know I'm still a valid member of society rather than a freak of nature. Yes, even those people I don't necessarily like. But I'm working on that...

6. CROHNED TO PERFECTION: YOU ARE STRONGER THAN YOU THINK

Try to think back to how you were pre-Crohn's. No, I'm not trying some bizarre hypnotherapy; I can't cure you via the written word. For that you have to call 08500-300-567 and pay £60 per minute for my words of wisdom (always remember to ask the bill payer's permission before dialling). The reason I say this is to remind you what sort of person you were before and just how far you've come. For me, I didn't like needles; who does though? I wasn't by any means phobic, but injections were certainly not moments I relished. Now, I don't even flinch when a syringe is stuck in my arm. Or when there are tubes and needles sticking out of/in every available orifice. It's easier now, because I've had to accept the fact that it's part of my life. I didn't think pre-Crohn's that I'd have been able to cope with all the tests and procedures I've been through, but I have. That doesn't mean I've skipped in my nightie towards an MRI scanner, guzzling the bowel prep with glee, but it does mean I've learned to listen much more carefully and intently to what is about to happen to me. If it happens to be something I don't, or won't like, I grit my teeth and get it over with. With every hospital visit I feel braver and bolder than ever before.

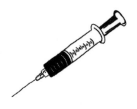

7. SKIN AND CROHN'S: BODY TALKS

I've gained a much greater understanding of the inner workings of my body. I've become knowledgeable in areas of medicine I hitherto didn't have the first clue about. I've learned to understand the effects of different drugs and treatments and the impact they have on my health.

When living with a chronic illness it's vital you make yourself aware of what your body can handle. Think of your body as a car; you wouldn't leave the house in a vehicle without filling it up with petrol, so don't start your day without having breakfast. Fuel yourself. Try to ensure you educate yourself on what the disease means for you and the future running of your body.

Forewarned is forearmed. Soak up all you can from the doctors and learn some about your tum.

Educating yourself on Crohn's, and doing your own research outside the doctors' surgery, can be a minefield. Stick to questioning your consultants and specialists and boning up on any literature they provide or can recommend. Initially try to steer clear of websites and books unless they have an unbiased and impartial view. Excluding this one of course.

8. THE GUTTY PROFESSOR: LISTEN TO YOUR BODY

This is a very important tool that most patients gain shortly after diagnosis. So far you've reached this stage of your life by listening to your gut (literally) when it was viciously telling you to sort yourself out, rudely forcing you to the toilet or coldly knocking you out, so continue to heed these warnings. Pay attention to symptoms and anything you feel may be out of the ordinary, and don't let anything escalate; if you are worried, see a doctor. Yes it might well be nothing, but it's *something*, and it's that something that's worried you enough to consider getting checked out, so do it. *Go with your gut instinct.* It's always better to be safe than sorry, and you alone know when things are off kilter.

In my case, the main signs I'm approaching a flare-up are excessive and continued diarrhoea, grumbling stomach, dry skin, ulcers/cold sores, aching joints and niggling or intense and prolonged pain in my stomach and lower back. All of these things happen most days, nothing out of the ordinary, but now when they all act up together, like the world's worst performance, I (try to) stand up and take notice. Your body has a megaphone inside it screaming out to be heard, so open your ears from time to time.

9. YOU CROHNLY LIVE ONCE: BE OPEN TO CHANGE

Depending on your personality pre-disease, this may be harder for some than others. This illness can be incredibly limiting in the things you can do and plans you can make. Crohnie's can't really plan in advance, because we literally don't know how we will feel from one minute to the next. I can get up feeling great, have a tiny cup of tea and suddenly find myself floored and in agony for anything from a few hours to the rest of the day. Not ideal. Also, not very easy to explain to friends when you are forced to cancel plans or reschedule at the last minute.

I've had: 'But you were fine this morning/yesterday/ last week.' You're not really getting it are you?

I've been accused of 'playing the Crohn's card' in order to get out of things. A phrase that is both unbelievably ignorant and supremely insulting in equal measure.

With Crohn's you have to be realistic and think carefully before committing yourself about whether you are physically able to do certain things. It's difficult and frustrating but has to be done for your own sake and that of those around you. Loved ones won't care if you miss a dinner or don't feel up to staying out late; they will understand. The bottom line (pun, as always, intended) is that your health is paramount. Partying can always wait till you can comfortably squeeze your arthritic ankles into those six-inch heels.

10. THROW ME AN INTESTINE: APPLY PERSPECTIVE

This is another valuable lesson Crohn's has taught me. I've learned to try to change the way I see things and then how I deal with them. I focus on the big problems, rather than making small ones bigger. I don't allow myself to get stressed, as I know it will only serve to exacerbate my symptoms.

Life is too short to worry about the 'what ifs'. Spending so much time in hospital and away from loved ones has made me realise just how important it is that I make the most of the time I do have. Getting worked up about problems that are minor in the grand scheme of things, or issues outwith my control, is truly pointless. If I've got a lot on my mind, I try to list mentally my worries in order of priority. What's the most important issue and what can be done about it? What can't wait? Then I take it one at a time. Don't overload yourself with concerns. You are not superhuman. Can anyone take some of the pressure off? Ask them.

Concentrate on what really matters and don't let anything distract you from feeling as well as you can.

CROHN OF THE BRAVE

When experiencing a period of serious, debilitating and perhaps even life-threatening illness or, like myself, suffering from a chronic and incurable illness, there's a 99 per cent chance you'll have been referred to at some point as 'brave'. Let me first clarify that there's absolutely nothing wrong with that. It's a lovely word and its connotations are flattering in the extreme.

But why 'brave'?

Myself, as you know, I was diagnosed with Crohn's Disease, I got sick and got surgery, got a little better, then got sick again (repeat to infinity). I had no choice in any of it. I just had to grimace and bear it. Perhaps that's why this idea of 'bravery' is such a bugbear for me, because it's all outwith my control. I don't particularly WANT to have to be 'brave' or 'inspiring' or any other similes raided from the Thesaurus of Hallmark.

I WANT to be 'NORMAL'.

I don't consider myself brave, because I didn't choose this life. The Crohn's life chose me. I didn't decide to jump in front of a car to save a pensioner from getting thrown to their death. I didn't punch a shark in the face to stop it eating a child's leg. Or pull a morbidly obese man from a burning building wearing a gasoline-soaked maxi dress. I didn't even leave the last Jaffa Cake in the packet for SOMEONE ELSE to eat. All of these things, I consider acts of bravery – bold moves performed out of choice. Selfless acts to benefit someone else. Placing *yourself* at risk, without consideration. I *'put myself at risk'* when I take medication that gives me horrible side effects, when I go under the surgeon's knife or use a public toilet in a train station. But I didn't choose to be 'brave'. I chose to accept my lot and get on with it. Because really, what is my alternative? Play the martyr? Die? Where's the bravery in that?

I suppose I dislike this idea of being thought of as 'brave' mainly because I often don't feel it. What's brave about squirming every time you think about getting examined or squeezing the bottom of the chair when you get another blood test? I regularly feel weak and powerless and that I have no choice but to bow down to my illness. That makes me frustrated, angry and certainly not someone who would 'inspire' anything other than pitiful glances.

I feel at my bravest when I tell you that I don't feel brave. I often feel anything but. Bravery comes from making the absolute best of yourself *in spite* of an illness. Attitude is everything. You are limited in your choices so choose wisely; choose to be happy.

Now that's inspirational.

TO EACH HIS CROHN

So the end is almost nigh for this humble wee tale. Now we face the final colon. It's time for us all to look towards the future.

Although this book must inevitably come to an end, it doesn't mark the end of my, or any other Crohn's sufferer's, story.

This disease, as I *may* have mentioned 4,548,783,157,841 times previously, is, unfortunately, incurable. So, if no cure is found in my lifetime, I will, at the very least, have this strange bedfellow with me along for the rest of my earthly ride.

I've accepted my disease. As much as one can, I imagine.

Having Crohn's Disease has changed my life entirely and in immeasurable ways. Not completely for the worse, I should add. It has been, and I suppose always will be, a constant physical and mental challenge. It has forced me to re-evaluate what's truly important to me and whom I can rely on when times get tough and has introduced me to hundreds of new and incredible people I am now privileged enough to count as friends. The condition has educated me tenfold on my own weird and wonderful body and those of others. It's shown me what truly matters in life: love, health and happiness. It's helped me stop stressing about every little, inane, thing and focus on issues actually worth worrying about.

Having this illness has helped me communicate, coherently, with others, as to what's happening to my body. It's given me the confidence to talk to doctors and nurses without feeling ashamed, or embarrassed, about my medical trials. It's given me guts (and taken some away), colossal strength and the confidence to aim for my goals secure in the knowledge I will do my utmost not to let my illness stand in my way.

I've learned a million and one lessons and am sure I will keep on learning until my gas finally comes to a peep.

I love my illness in a strange (and possibly warped) way. I suppose I'm a lover not a fighter when it comes to Crohn's. Don't get me wrong, as I've said in no uncertain terms, it's a pretty volatile relationship, and I'm not entirely sure it loves me back *just yet*, but I'm working on that.

My disease has taught me an amazing amount about my own body. About everyone's body for that matter. About how amazingly, and mind-bogglingly well, they function (or not as the case may be).

It's been a thrilling adventure for a lassie such as me, who was once embarrassingly squeamish at the sight of her own nail breaking. Actually, that one still makes my stomach churn.

I've been through so many toe-curling procedures, and had so many implements inserted into so many orifices since then, I've just had to (wo)man up and get over that former girlish nausea. But enough about my weekend.

Crohn's Disease has made me acutely aware of what I can achieve if I set my mind to it. When you choose to accept your lot, and ensure you don't allow anger, bitterness and self-pity to eat you up, having this disease can fill you with a determination that's hard to fake. When your own body tries to set limits for you, that's when your mind puts its proverbial foot down and forces you to take action.

I've surprised myself in what I can cope with, and have already coped with, and how much I'm capable of when I really push myself. That, itself, can be a sliding scale, depending on the severity of your condition at any given time. Say somewhere between writing a book about it during a flare-up and climbing the stairs without almost passing out with exhaustion.

My love for my illness grows daily. I detest it and adore it in equal measure. I love to hate it, as Erasure once, wonderfully, put it. Not sure they were writing about bowel disease but a girl can dream. Much like an evening coming home from work to see dishes *still* piled in the sink from the night before, Crohn's disappoints me on a regular basis. Mild irritations and bugbears, as with any relationship, are a common occurrence, but you must learn to accept and find ways to make the best of, or even better, the situation. I've tried to look more in depth and focus on the positive sides of my illness. For me those 'benefits' are incredible. The brilliant friends I've made, the myriad knowledge I've gained and the amazing people I've somehow helped with my oft-blabbering writing, amongst others.

Chronic illness is an awful pain, quite literally, but also a constant reminder of how strong and resilient you can be.

I'm absolutely not trying to fool you into thinking that having Crohn's Disease is a 'good' thing. It's not. It's very hard and a daily challenge. You often feel your own body is conspiring against you. The breakthrough, though, comes with acceptance – knowing you can't change what's outwith your control but clinging on to what you can control and making the absolute most of the life you *still have*.

The main reason I've been reliving all this literal pain and heartache for you is not to be maudlin and self-pitying but to reiterate to any of you lovely readers that there are always going to be trials in your life, however small or insignificant they may seem compared with others, and you will always be tested. How you deal with those tests is truly in your hands. You can allow yourself to lie down to the challenges in your life and let yourself be steamrollered into the ground, or you can choose to be bolder than you thought possible and face these potentially tough times with enthusiasm and hope.

In the last few years I've been blogging and writing this book, it's become apparent that many of you actually *enjoy* reading my writing. Being Scottish and therefore practically incapable of accepting a compliment, this in itself is a bold move for me to admit. I've discovered how much I love writing, my Crohn's blog in particular. It's like a public diary for me (without all the explicit stuff, and by that obviously I mean how many Jaffa Cakes I can eat in one sitting) and in a way a form of therapy. To know many of you feel as I do, diseased or not, serves to remind me I'm not wholly insane. Or alone.

So I suppose I just really want to leave you with a reminder of the same thing. My wonderful friends and family have shown me in the last few years since my diagnosis that I am truly loved. It feels really good to be reminded, because sometimes it's just necessary. However much of a tough cookie you think you are.

I want to spread some of that warmth your way. Whoever you are, you are not alone, the feelings you feel are real and things are genuinely never as bad as they seem. There is always someone willing to listen if you are willing to talk. Open up and let someone in. I mean that in the least sexual way imaginable of course.

My dad might still be reading this.

(And it's 12 by the way – 12 bloody DELICIOUS Jaffa Cakes. Possibly my proudest achievement to date.)

I do truly hope that if you have this disease yourself, or even if you willingly care for a loved one who does, you will try to remember that even in the darkest of depths, and the bluest of moods, throughout the toughest of challenges there is *always* a light at the end of the colon. Even if it flickers and seems faint, and the bulb is about to burn out, it's still there. You just have to get up and look for it. Maybe jiggle it back into place a wee bit, as the actress said to the bishop.

After all, you have *Crohn's Disease*, you could take on a team of sumo-wrestling, boxing-trained, karate-expert ninjas and not even so much as break into a sweat.

Not literally of course! Or at the very least, only on the doctor's advice.

Whatever you do, don't listen to ME! I don't have the first clue what I'm doing. Why don't you pick up a self-help book or something?

6

NONSENSE

GIN AND CROHNIC

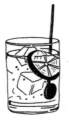

Before I bid you all a heartbreaking farewell, I still have a few pages in which to squeeze some miscellaneous nonsense. I've taken the liberty of compiling a few sections you may find useful as you or your loved ones head out into the world with your disease in tow.

DR STRANGELOVE

It's very important when you are first diagnosed to ensure you don't pile too much pressure on yourself. Finding out you or a loved one have IBD can be an incredibly upsetting, frightening and downright intimidating time. This is heightened if you have absolutely no knowledge of the ins and, more importantly, outs of your new illness. Forearmed is definitely forewarned but be careful not to focus too much on loading yourself with information from all angles. Start at the beginning and ask your doctor what the main issues that YOU will face are. Remember that no one with Crohn's is exactly the same, and what may work for you won't necessarily do the trick for the woman in the next bed.

It can be so overwhelming to learn of your diagnosis that it's hard to know what to ask. You'll find yourself leaving the doctor's office confused and a little dazed at the barrage of facts and figures he or she has laid out in front of you. Do not fear, for I have taken the liberty of compiling a few questions you may want to ask when you have your one on one with the medical professionals.

'WHAT TYPE OF IBD DO I HAVE, EXACTLY?'

This is relevant, as IBD can be separated into two separate medical conditions: Crohn's Disease or Ulcerative Colitis. These conditions fall under the same IBD umbrella, as they share issues in common. They affect the same/similar areas of the body and can both cause the same difficulty in reaching a diagnosis. It's vital you are aware from the get-go which of the two you will be dealing with, as, although they share characteristics, they are very different. In order to begin your own research you must know what you are looking for.

'WHAT SYMPTOMS SHOULD I LOOK OUT FOR/WORRY ABOUT?'

There are so many varied and wide-reaching symptoms of the condition that it's hard to pinpoint which should be concerning or which should be managed without the need for the emergency room. Your doctor should be able to explain what issues may be a cause for concern in your case. Don't worry if any of it sounds horrifying; it is their job to lay out all the facts – it doesn't necessarily mean any of it will happen to you. If it makes you feel more secure, insist you have a contact from the hospital/ your local surgery who you can reach easily if there is an emergency. This should serve as part of your treatment plan from the outset.

'WILL I EVER BE CURED?'

Your doctor should make this clear from the beginning, however unfortunately in many cases patients can be left under the impression that following treatment or surgery they will no longer have the disease. This misconception generally comes more from the media, word of mouth and misleading articles than medical professionals, mind you. It's disheartening to discover that you have an 'incurable' illness, but it also allows you to face up to the fact that you will have to knuckle down and focus on adapting to your new life. The alternative is living a life of 'waiting to get better', which is really no life at all.

'WILL I END UP WITH OTHER CONDITIONS AS A RESULT OF IBD?'

This may be challenging to predict, so don't assume if you ask your doctor this question and they have difficulty in answering it that they are trying to withhold anything from you. Each patient reacts to medication differently and each patient will adapt to their condition in their own way. Other issues can show themselves months or years down the line following on from an IBD diagnosis, but if you want to allow yourself some background knowledge before the event then your consultant should be able to give you a bit of an early-warning system.

'WHAT SHOULD I DO TO HELP MYSELF?'

A great question this one, and one that normally gets brownie points galore from the medical professionals. They just LOVE to see you taking responsibility for your own health and not sitting down to illness. On the whole, this is encouraging and shows that you are looking to a silver lining despite having Crohn's. It's also a very positive outlook – only you know your own body and what works – essentially you will be the one living with this on a daily basis so any tips and tricks of the trade you can learn to make life easier are always as welcome as a bumper pack of toilet roll.

ACHE IT LIKE A POLAROID PICTURE

It can be scary being out in the world and outwith your comfort zone with a chronic condition. The simple idea of not knowing where the nearest bathroom is can send a patient into a mild state of panic. One of the most important aspects of living with Crohn's is ensuring, wherever possible, that *you* are in control – of your illness and your bowels. So, almost like I'd planned it, here I have compiled a few phrases you may find useful if you find yourself jetting across the globe with your Crohn's Disease along for the ride!

(The last one is a personal choice of mine following a horrific incident in Barcelona 2008 from which the maid of the Grand Hotel bathroom probably hasn't fully recovered.)

'WHERE IS THE TOILET?'

- '¿Dónde está el baño?' (Spanish)

- 'Où sont les toilettes?' (French)

- 'Onde é o banheiro?' (Portuguese)

- 'Waar is het toilet?' (Dutch)

- 'Wo ist die Toilette?' (German)

- 'Dov'è il bagno?' (Italian)

'WHERE IS THE NEAREST HOSPITAL?'

- '¿Dónde está el hospital más cercano?' (Spanish)

- 'Où est l'hôpital le plus proche?' (French)

- 'Onde está o hospital mais próximo?' (Portuguese)

- 'Waar is het dichtstbijzijnde ziekenhuis?' (Dutch)

- 'Wo ist das nächste Krankenhaus?' (German)

- 'Dove si trova l'ospedale più vicino?' (Italian)

'WHERE IS THE NEAREST PHARMACY?'

- '¿Dónde está la farmacia más cercana?' (Spanish)

- 'Où se trouve la pharmacie la plus proche?' (French)

- 'Onde fica a farmácia mais próxima?' (Portuguese)

- 'Waar is de dichtstbijzijnde apotheek?' (Dutch)

- 'Wo ist die nächste Apotheke?' (German)

- 'Dove si trova la farmacia più vicina?' (Italian)

'I HAVE A CHRONIC MEDICAL CONDITION'

- 'Tengo una condición médica crónica.' (Spanish)

- 'J'ai un problème de santé chronique.' (French)

- 'Eu tenho uma condição médica crônica.' (Portuguese)

- 'Ik heb een chronische medische aandoeningen.' (Dutch)

- 'Ich habe einen chronischen Erkrankungen.' (German)

- 'Ho un condizioni mediche croniche.' (Italian)

'I REQUIRE MEDICAL ATTENTION'

- 'I requieren atención médica.' (Spanish)

- 'J'ai besoin d'une attention médicale.' (French)

- 'I requerem atenção médica.' (Portuguese)

- 'Ik medische zorg nodig.' (Dutch)

- 'I benötigen medizinische Versorgung.' (German)

- 'Ho bisogno di cure mediche.' (Italian)

'COULD YOU REPLACE THE TOILET ROLL?'

- '¿Podría reemplazar el rollo de papel higiénico?' (Spanish)

- 'Pourriez-vous remplacer le rouleau de papier toilette?' (French)

- 'Você poderia substituir o rolo de papel higiénico?' (Portuguese)

- 'Kunt u de toiletrol te vervangen?' (Dutch)

- 'Könnten Sie den WC-Rollen ersetzen?' (German)

- 'Potresti sostituire il rotolo di carta igienica?' (Italian)

'PLEASE TELL ME THERE ARE NO CHILLIES IN THIS?'

- '¿Por favor me dice que no hay chiles en esto?' (Spanish)

- 'S'il vous plaît dites-moi, il n'y a pas de piments dans cette?' (French)

- 'Por favor me diga que não há pimentões neste?' (Portuguese)

- 'Kunt u mij zeggen dat er geen chilipepers in deze?' (Dutch)

- 'Bitte sagen Sie mir, es gibt keine Chilischoten in das?' (German)

- 'La prego di dirmi non ci sono peperoncini in questo?' (Italian)

RAGE AGAINST THE LATRINE

I started this final section with the idea of attempting to compile a few of my own nuggets of advice in coping with Crohn's (see below), but then I had a minor lightbulb moment. Who better to share their own insight and words of wisdom on this very subject than the sufferers themselves?!

I began my intense and unrelenting research by asking my Facebook friends and Twitter and blog followers what tips they could share and what they find invaluable when living with their Crohn's Disease. The outcome was a pool of diseased wisdom I could fish in for days! So here are a few of my own catches and a few of my favourites of *yours* slipped in the net too!

It was *THIS BIG*!

(**Thank you** to all who contributed!)

'Like dogs and diamonds before them, you will discover that wet wipes are now your best friend.'

'Reduce your stress and eat better. Of course, exponentially easier said than done!'

@boydacus

'Learning to control your breathing is a good way to distract yourself from pain. Since you've asked, my personal choice is Stayin' Alive by the Bee Gees as my go-to song to help me focus my breathing. Funkiness personified with an apt title.'

'"Look good, feel better" no matter how bad I am feeling I always put a face on. I don't want to look like death even if I feel it!'

J. Ziolkowski

'Don't discount any minor pains or strange goings on at your rear as nothing. If need be document any issues as they happen so you have a solid (or not so as the case may be...) record of your symptoms. Take this, and yourself, to the doctor if you are concerned.'

'Remember to keep hydrated if you can't eat.'

S. O'Brien

'Keep a food diary. Log everything you eat and drink and how you feel before and after meals. This is a great way to track what your Crohn's can and can't tolerate, and can help you plan your diet around your disease.'

'Maintain your sense of humour whenever possible.'

G. Barratt

'Learn as much as you can about your condition. It's your body; knowledge is power.'

'When your life revolves around hospitals and doctors' surgeries, it's great to focus on something outside of it all – take up a hobby – enjoy nature and concentrate on the good in your life, it works wonders.'

C. & J. Clark

'Be as honest and open as you can with doctors and nurses. They are genuinely un-shockable and need to know about your backside to be able help you! Now is your chance to talk about it! Grab that chance with both paws!'

'Speak up to your doctors and don't let them push you around. Never take meds you aren't comfortable with.'

@octofussy

'Difficulty in getting across exactly how you feel to the doctor? Write everything down. This allows you to think clearly and not get distracted or confused by medical jargon.'

'A wheat bag is good for easing low-level tummy pain.'

L. F. Macmillan

'If you feel awkward explaining your disease to new people, for example at a party, take a roll of toilet paper. Explain briefly you have Crohn's Disease and may have to use their toilet more than most. It's an icebreaker that allows the potential awkwardness of leaving the room later in the night to dissipate before it's even formed.'

'Know that you are never the only one going through this.'

V. Laine

'Make sure you keep talking – don't hide away, and be open and honest with those who love you, as they want and need to know.'

'Wherever you are in the world, always have your eye on the toilet signs.'

@LesterThompson1

GLOSSARY

WIPING AWAY THE MYTHS

I truly hope you've enjoyed my tales of diseased debauchery. However, if you've found yourself baffled by any of the medical terminology I've used, or just want to learn a little more about a Crohn's patient's body, then you can spy on me whilst I'm undressing or (and my preferred choice) you could peruse the following glossary of bottom-related belters to further your knowledge.

ANUS — the anus is the external opening of the rectum, where the gastrointestinal (GI) tract ends.

APPENDICITIS — a serious medical condition, normally requiring urgent medical intervention, in which the appendix becomes inflamed and incredibly painful.

APPENDIX — a thin tube about four inches long that sits at the junction of the small intestine and large intestine. Generally the appendix sits in the lower right abdomen, and its function is still unknown.

ARTHRITIS — a joint disorder that involves inflammation of more than one joint.

B12 – one of the eight 'B' vitamins with a key role in the normal functioning of the brain and nervous system and the formation of blood.

COLON – the large intestine (the colon) is the last part of the digestive system. Its function is to absorb water from the remaining indigestible food matter and then to expel useless waste material from the body. Unlike the small intestine, the colon does not play a major role in absorption of foods and nutrients. However, it does absorb water, sodium and some fat-soluble vitamins. The colon consists of four sections: the ascending colon, the traverse colon, the descending colon and the sigmoid colon.

COLONOSCOPY – the endoscopic examination of the large bowel and part of the small bowel with a Charge-Coupled Device (CCD) camera or a fibre-optic camera on a flexible tube passed through the anus. It provides visual results and can help with diagnosis. Often biopsies are taken throughout the procedure for testing.

COLOSTOMY (BAG) – prosthetic medical device providing a means for the collection of waste from a 'surgically diverted' biological system, and the creation of a stoma.

CONSTIPATION – where there is difficulty in emptying the bowels, usually associated with hardened faeces.

CORTISONE INJECTIONS — these are used to help treat several issues including bursitis, tendonitis and arthritis, amongst other words ending in 'itis'. Corticosteroid injections are also used for conditions such as allergic reactions and asthma.

CROHN'S DISEASE — really?! Have you learnt nothing?! Ok. It is an incurable condition that causes inflammation of the lining of the digestive system. It most commonly occurs in the small or large intestine, but can affect any part of the digestive system from mouth to anus. The most common symptoms of the disease include abdominal pain, weight loss, diarrhoea, extreme fatigue and blood in the stool.

DAVID BOWIE — God.

DIARRHOEA — the passing of watery stools that is more than normal for you, generally associated with an infection or longstanding illness.

DIGESTIVE SYSTEM — the purpose of the digestive system is to help the body digest food. This part of the body is made up of the GI tract (see above), liver, pancreas and gallbladder. These are the solid organs of the digestive system. Bacteria in the GI tract help with digestion; together with a combination of nerves, blood, hormones and the aforementioned organs, the digestive system completes the complex task of digesting the foods and drinks we consume daily.

ENDOSCOPY – procedure whereby the inside of the body is examined using an endoscope, which is a thin, flexible tube with a video camera attached at the end. Images are relayed to a screen to aid diagnosis. The endoscope is inserted into the body through the throat, anus or even a small insertion made into the skin.

FAECAL CALPROTECTIN – a test carried out from a patient's stool sample to establish the range/level of inflammation. Ranges vary dependent on age, however generally in IBD sufferers 0–50 = normal, 51–120 = borderline and 120+ = abnormal.

FAECAL MATTER – solid excretory product evacuated from the bowels.

FAECES – the waste product of the human digestive system; also referred to as stool.

GASTROINTESTINAL (GI) TRACT – also known as the digestive tract, the GI tract is a series of hollow organs joined together through a long and snaking tube from the mouth to the anus. The organs that make up the GI tract are the mouth, oesophagus, stomach, small intestine, large intestine (including the rectum) and anus. Food enters the mouth and passes to the anus through these organs within the GI tract.

INFLAMMATORY BOWEL DISEASE (IBD) – this is a term mainly used to describe two diseases: Ulcerative Colitis (UC) and Crohn's Disease. Both UC and Crohn's are long-term (chronic) diseases that most prominently involve inflammation of the gastrointestinal tract. UC only affects the colon, while Crohn's Disease can affect the entire digestive system from the mouth to the anus. It can often be difficult to tell the difference between the two main types of IBD. In these cases, it's known as 'indeterminate colitis'. Much rarer types of IBD exist called 'collagenous colitis' and 'lymphocytic colitis'. Together these are often called 'microscopic colitis'.

INFUSION – this involves the administration of medication through a needle or catheter. It is generally prescribed when a patient's condition cannot be treated effectively by oral medications. It is particularly useful for IBD patients who have difficulty with absorption.

INTESTINES – these are vital organs within the GI tract of the digestive system. Their functions are to digest food and enable nutrients that food releases to enter into the body's bloodstream. They consist of the small and large intestine.

IRRITABLE BOWEL SYNDROME (IBS) – this is a common condition affecting the digestive system. It can cause bouts of stomach cramps, bloating, diarrhoea and constipation.

MERCAPTOPURINE — an immunosuppressive medication. Occasionally known as 6-MP. It is commonly used to treat Crohn's Disease and Ulcerative Colitis, particularly after resection surgery. It has also been known to treat acute lymphocytic leukaemia either used alone or with other chemotherapy drugs.

MORPHINE — an opiate drug used in treating chronic and acute pain. It can be given in many forms and by many different methods. The medication has a high tendency to be addictive therefore is generally not used in the long term.

OSTOMY — an artificial opening in an organ of the body created during an operation such as a colostomy, ileostomy or gastrostomy; a stoma which comes from the Greek word for 'mouth' or 'opening'.

RECTUM — the lower part of the large intestine, which holds stool until it is expelled.

RESECTION — a surgical procedure to remove part of an organ or gland. It may also be used to remove a tumour and normal tissue around it.

SEDATIVE — also commonly referred to as a tranquilliser, this is a substance that induces sedation by reducing irritability or excitement. When provided in higher doses it can cause slurred speech, dizziness and unreliable reflexes.

SIGMOIDOSCOPY — a procedure used to see inside the sigmoid colon and rectum.

STEROIDS — sometimes called a 'corticosteroid' this medication treats a variety of problems. It is commonly used in the initial treatment of IBD or during flare-ups of the condition, as it reduces inflammation and affects the immune system.

STOOL — the waste product of the human digestive system; also referred to as faeces.

ULCERATIVE COLITIS (UC) — a form of IBD that causes long-lasting inflammation and ulcers (sores) in the digestive tract. It usually affects the innermost lining of the large intestine and rectum. UC can be debilitating and can often lead to life-threatening complications.

THE (REAR) END

ACKNOWLEDGEMENTS

This book wouldn't have been in any way possible, if it wasn't for the encouragement and enthusiasm *you* have had for my writing. Absolutely everyone who has taken the time to read my blog has bolstered my knowledge and confidence in ways I never thought possible. THANK YOU.

My family and friends have never faltered in their support and understanding of my illness from day one. My mum, Kathleen, and dad, Richard, have been with me every step of the way, with unfaltering encouragement, love and support. They are the most amazing parents I could ever have and I'm proud to call myself their daughter. I love you both so much my heart could burst out of my chest. What with my existing medical conditions, that could prove testing, so I hope writing it down here is sufficient enough for you.

My (unofficial) in-laws Mary and Peter, and Angela and her beautiful girls, have shown me the kindness and love of a whole other family into which they have welcomed me with open arms (and a sick bowl where necessary). They have been tireless with their willingness to take me to and from the hospital and, more importantly, their compassion.

My 'wee' brother Mark has been a fountain of knowledge on the scary world of writing a book and a revelation in his ability to make his sister feel like the most important person in the world.

The love I have for you all is boundless.

Special mention to my incredibly wonderful friends too – if I've forgotten anyone I apologise, but this isn't a bloody Oscar speech, *get over it.*

Sarah (always the best and brightest cow in my field), Nichola (forever and always Grannies fo' Life), Jen (hope we're still 'smelling the basil' together when we are pensioners, Dale), Sam (the pâté to my oatcakes), Nicola and Collette (the best bosses to turn into friends ever), Nicola J (my lover from another mother), Lisa (keeping it 'phat with me since Primary 1), Lyndsay (always making my 'tash curl with happiness), Megan (my back passage never knew the meaning of clean till I met you), Kate (I'd love to have the words like Wild-Eyes to create a special card just for you), Karen (I hope you'll always be on hand to dance for me when I can't), Deanna (you've shown me strength to aspire to), Angela (you're the kindest most wonderful sister from another mister), Ariadna (you taught me that 'cagada' means poop in Spanish and so much more) – you have all helped me cope in your own unique and intuitive ways.

You have never allowed me to wallow, made me laugh, let me cry (for an inordinate amount of time), wiped my tears (and thankfully nothing else… yet), let me talk and shown me what friendship truly means. I adore all of you spectacularly and am unbelievably lucky to have you all in my life.

Special thanks to John Bradley for his writing expertise and helping me conquer my fear of public speaking (sort of), and all of the amazing people who live inside my phone who are always on hand for advice and support!

James, you are, and continue to be, the cheese to my macaroni. You make me laugh till it hurts and make me feel I can achieve anything I set my mind to. You truly are my better half. You are the best and most delicious medicine I prescribe for myself.

OH, and of course the cats!

Dupin and Khan you are the furriest little bundles of love a cat-lady could ask for – the best wee cuddly nurses ever! And all cats in general, thanks for being SO CUTE. Get your owners to read this to you in between petting sessions.

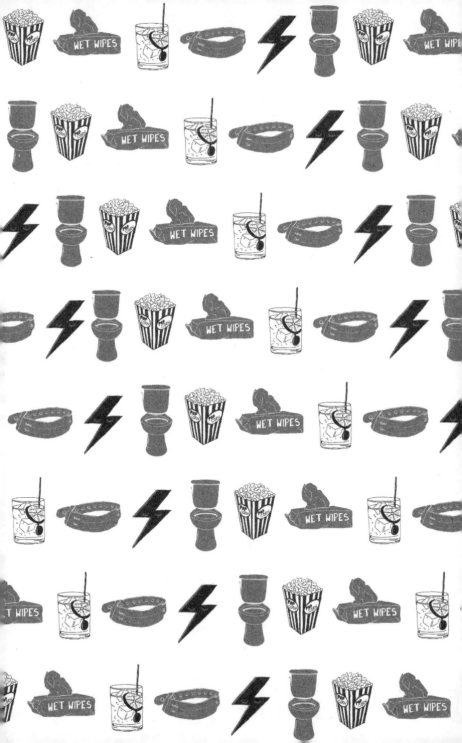

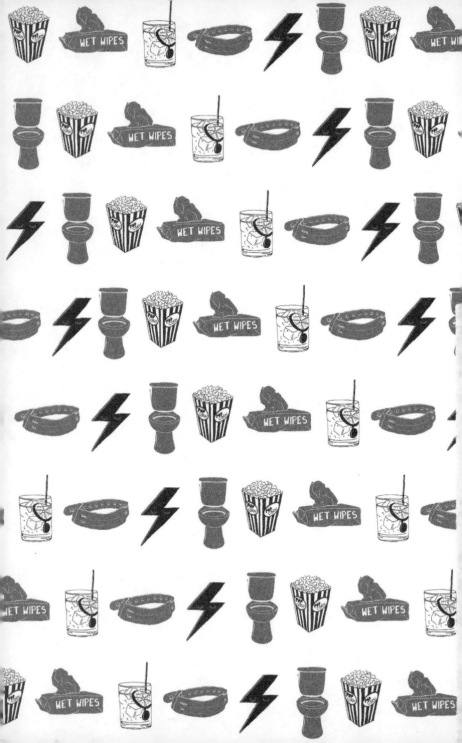